Why Yoga Works

&

How It Can Work For You

WHY YOGA WORKS
&
HOW IT CAN WORK FOR YOU

Based on the Teachings of T. Krishnamacharya and T.K.V. Desikachar

Robert Birnberg, Christine Dormaier & Fran Ubertini

2018

MEDICAL DISCLAIMER

All information in this book is to be used at your own discretion and, if possible, under the guidance of a qualified teacher.

All techniques and practices are meant to serve as a complement rather than a substitute for medical care. We strongly recommend that you consult with a licensed health care professional before attempting any of the practices in this book.

First published in USA in 2018 by Robert Birnberg, Christine Dormaier & Fran Ubertini

Printed in the USA

Library of Congress Control Number: 2018909882

ISBN-10:0692096892

ISBN-13:978-0692096895 (Yoga Unites FRC, LLC)

Published by Yoga Unites Publications, Seattle, Washington

WhyYogaWorks.com

Ordering Information: Special discounts are available on quantity purchases. For details, contact Sales@WhyYogaWorks.com.

Book design, layout & cover art: Andres Adamson - www.andresadamson.com

Copy editor: Wayne Lee - www.wayneleepoet.com

We would like to dedicate this book

to our life partners

Eleni, Tim and Tom.

Table Of Contents

Acknowledgements

As the authors, we have discovered that self-publishing is a uniquely arduous process that requires the skills and support of a few gifted experts in their fields. We would like to acknowledge the handful of extraordinary people from around the world who have helped make our book a reality.

Our thanks go out to Andres Adamson in Pärnu, Estonia, for his creative formatting and for transforming our ideas into beautiful illustrations; Jessica McCurdy-Crooks in Kingston, Jamaica, for her detailed attention to our index; Judy Bentley in Seattle, Washington, for her keen proofreading, Aja Thomas in Portland, Oregon, for his Sanskrit expertise; and special thanks to Wayne Lee, another Oregonian, our patient editor, who was instrumental in helping us find our voice.

And finally, we would like to express our heartfelt gratitude to our teacher, Sonia Nelson, for her guidance, support and clarity on the teachings presented in this book.

Foreword

From the teaching tradition of T. Krishnamacharya and T.K.V. Desikachar, the practice of *Yoga* can be seen as that which enables us to do something we could not do before. This principle can be applied to all aspects of life whether making our bodies stronger and more flexible, increasing the quality of our energy and capacity of our breathing, stabilizing and focusing our minds, clarifying and giving direction to our actions or creating more positive relationships.

In a rare coming together of diverse education, teaching experience and individual talents, Christine Dormaier, Fran Ubertini and Robert Birnberg have remarkably synthesized many years of dedicated study, practice and teaching. In authoring *Why Yoga Works*, they present an accessible vehicle for the intellectual understanding of *Yoga*'s fundamental principles and through a variety of skillfully designed practices, they provide an effective medium for understanding through concrete experience. Additionally, they have offered the necessary guidance for practicing outside the context of a group or individual class while encouraging the practitioner to go beyond the book itself by finding a teacher who can support their evolution on the path of *Yoga*.

Organized to easily find the sections that interest us most, *Why Yoga Works* brings us back again and again to deepen and refine our understanding and experience of one of the world's great *Yoga* traditions.

Sonia Nelson

INTRODUCTION

The Legacy of T. Krishnamacharya

Throughout *Yoga*'s long and rich history, there have been countless teachers, interpretations and applications of its core principles. Why *Yoga* Works & How it Can Work for You is inspired by the legacy of one of the most influential of these teachers, the South Indian *Yoga* master Śrī Tirumalai Krishnamacharya (1888-1989), known to the world simply as T. Krishnamacharya. His unique insights into the essence of *Yoga* were then handed down to his son, T.K.V. Desikachar (1938-2016), a world-class teacher, healer and innovator, who passed them on to us.

Over the past 20 years, we three co-authors were blessed to have attended his retreats, workshops and trainings throughout the world. Our dedicated study of these powerful teachings and one-on-one work with T.K.V. Desikachar's long-time students have transformed our lives and informed every aspect of our work as *Yoga* teachers, *Yoga* therapists and *Yoga* teacher trainers.

This book is born out of our desire to share these profound, life-changing teachings with you, whatever your background or experience. We have chosen to illustrate the practices with stick figures, as this is the method we use to design practices for our students and also to serve as a teaching tool for those wishing to draw practices for themselves or their students.

Perhaps you are someone who has just recently noticed *Yoga*'s widespread popularity and are curious about its benefits. Maybe you are a regular *Yoga* practitioner or even a *Yoga* teacher. No matter who you are or whatever your experience, this book will help you deepen your understanding of *Yoga*'s principles (Why *Yoga* Works) and give you the tools to practice this ancient healing art yourself (How It Can Work for You). All Sanskrit words in this book, including *Yoga*, are italicized. For clarification they are defined in the Glossary of Sanskrit Terms.

In Part I (Why *Yoga* Works) you will learn about the 5,000-year history and foundation of this holistic system. We will delve into *Yoga*'s underlying philosophy and explore its practical guidelines for enhancing personal growth and maintaining a balanced lifestyle.

In Part II (How It Can Work for You) we explore the use of movement, focused breath work and meditation. We explain how to create a *Yoga* practice tailored to your own individual needs, abilities and goals and offer detailed exercises, techniques and practices for you to try.

We wish you health, happiness and long life.

--RB, CD & FU

"The ultimate goal of *Yoga* is to always observe things accurately and therefore never act in a way that will make us regret our actions later."

T.K.V. Desikachar

PART I:

Why *Yoga* Works

CHAPTER 1

A Brief History of *Yoga*

In a world where health fads and self-help crazes come and go on a monthly basis, *Yoga* is as relevant today as it was 5,000 years ago. Even though technological advances seem to have improved our quality of living, humans worldwide continue to struggle with the same basic challenges of survival, maintaining health, finding happiness and cultivating truly satisfying relationships.

In Sanskrit, the word *Yoga* means "to join two or more things together" or "to link." *Yoga* is both a state of connection and a system of techniques for carefully joining the body, breath and mind, to create and maintain this linked state. For many modern practitioners, *Yoga* consists of being guided through a series of poses leading to a rest at the end. This emphasis on posture (*āsana*), rather than cultivating the complete integration of body, breath and mind, offers a fraction of the benefits that *Yoga* practice can have on the human system. One of the intentions of this book is to expand, refine and clarify this perception and to deepen your understanding of the full scope and depth of *Yoga*.

However you define it, *Yoga* is more popular now than at any time in history. The secret to *Yoga*'s ever-increasing popularity is that it is, and always has been, a powerful antidote to life's suffering (*duḥkha*). Today, some practitioners use *Yoga* to achieve greater flexibility, physical strength and stamina. Many practice to create mental stability and calmness. Others use *Yoga* therapeutically, to enhance individual wellness and to reduce the symptoms and causes of disease. Though *Yoga* is not a religion, it supports any existing spiritual or religious practice, as well as adding a new spiritual dimension to your life.

To fully understand *Yoga*'s enduring appeal, we must first explore its past. What we know as *Yoga* today has a rich history drawn from a variety of teachings, many of which are unfamiliar to the general public. This chapter provides a brief history of *Yoga*, along with an introduction to its basic terminology.

The *Vedas*

The *Vedas* are some of the most ancient wisdom teachings known to man. They are the result of special teachings "received" by great sages in their meditations. For more than 3,500 years, throughout the world, these great wisdom teachings have served as a multi-dimensional guide for living. They have been orally transmitted in the form of hymns, stories, poems and *mantras*. Though the four books of the *Vedas*: *Ṛg*, *Yajur*, *Sāma* and *Atharva*, are not widely studied in the west, they provide the foundation upon which *Yoga* is based.

The *Upaniṣads*

In the post-*Vedic* period (800-300 BCE), the world witnessed dramatic religious and philosophical changes. In an attempt to make the *Vedas* more accessible, the philosophers of that time presented a new body of knowledge, the *Upaniṣads* (to sit near). Though today we study these teachings through written texts, the *Upaniṣads* were originally presented as dialogues between teacher and student and offered a broad range of practical tools for living.

The *Upaniṣads* are the source of many of *Yoga*'s core concepts, including *dhyāna* (meditation), *prāṇa* (life force), *śraddhā* (the concept of faith and conviction) and the importance of a student/teacher relationship.

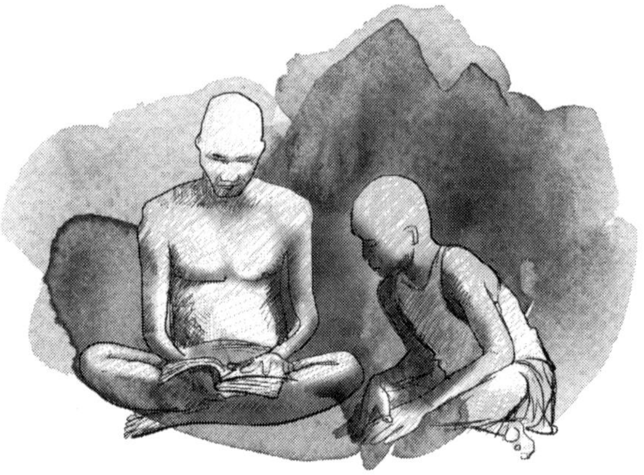

The *Bhagavad Gītā*

The *Bhagavad Gītā*, "the Song of the Beloved," was written sometime between the second century BCE and the fifth century CE. It is considered to be one of the most important philosophical teachings in history, revered as both a sacred text of Hinduism and a primary reference for *Yoga*.

Made up of 700 verses, the *Bhagavad Gītā* is part of a larger epic story, the *Mahābhārata*. The format is an extended conversation between a teacher, Krishna, and his student, Arjuna. It covers such fundamental topics as duty, morality, nonattachment and devotion. This timeless, practical manual for daily living has influenced such diverse historical figures as Mahātma Gandhi, Albert Einstein and Henry David Thoreau.

The *Darśanas*

Despite the vast knowledge and wisdom contained in the *Vedas* and *Upaniṣads*, great sages were aware of humanity's ongoing pervasive suffering, as well as the need for practical tools to promote physical, psychological and social well-being. This realization led to the creation of six philosophical systems called the *Darśanas* (ways of looking at life): ***Nyāya, Vaiśeṣika, Sāṃkhya, Mīmāṃsā, Vedānta*** and ***Yoga***. The *Darśanas* offer six distinct paths to the common goal of identifying and reducing suffering. Though all six *Darśanas* are worthy of further study, this book will focus on *Sāṃkhya* and *Yoga*.

Sāṃkhya Darśana

Yoga's underlying view of reality is presented in the *Sāṃkhya Darśana*. An understanding of this ancient philosophy is essential to fully embrace *Yoga*'s breadth, depth and scope. *Sāṃkhya* is a description of evolution and nature, describing all reality as having two components, *puruṣa* (spirit) and *prakṛti* (matter). These two components exist in a symbiotic relationship. *Puruṣa* can only experience itself through *prakṛti*; without *puruṣa*, all matter is unconscious and inanimate.

Puruṣa is the formless, unchanging, individual consciousness at the core of our being, the part of us that observes our experiences and actions from the moment of birth until we die. This observer, like an inner GPS, is always guiding us (whether or not we are listening) toward where we should be and what we should be doing.

Prakṛti is the material world, whose form is constantly changing. It is all matter, including nature and the human body, as well as the mind with all its thoughts and emotions. Just as trees change with the seasons, the tides with the phases of the moon and our emotions throughout the day, transformation is the very essence of this component. *Prakṛti* has three energetic qualities, or varying degrees of change, called the *guṇas*.

The first *guṇa* is *rajas*, the quality of change which is intense, turbulent and dynamic. In the natural world, fire is an example of *rajas*. Where fire exists, form changes quickly: paper becomes ash, wood becomes ember, cool oxygen and organic matter become hot carbon dioxide. Humans often experience this *guṇa* as having the energy and motivation to complete tasks and achieve goals. It also presents as hyperactivity, anxiety, agitation, nervousness and insomnia.

The second *guṇa* is *tamas*, expressing qualities such as heaviness, dullness and resistance to change. In the natural world, rock is *tamasic* because it changes form, but slowly and only after much pressure is applied. Humans often experience *tamas* as stability and a good night's sleep. However, it is also responsible for fatigue, lethargy, doubt, hopelessness and depression.

Sattva, the third *guṇa,* is change that is harmonious, balanced and sustainable. An example of *sattva* in the natural world is a clear, calm pool of water. According to *Sāṃkhya*, though the mind moves between *rajas* and *tamas*, the unchanging characteristic of *puruṣa* can only be experienced by a *sattvic* mind. A mind that is too agitated (*rajasic*), or too dull (*tamasic*), only perceives its own movement and cannot know the inherent consciousness at its core.

In order to be stable, content and able to perceive our deepest truths, a *sattvic* mind is required. Therefore, based on *Sāṃkhya*, *Yoga*'s strategy for reducing suffering is cultivating and sustaining a *sattvic* mind.

Yoga Darśana: Patanjali's *Yoga Sūtras*

Though the word *Yoga* appears throughout the *Vedas,* it differs from the *Darśana* of *Yoga* which is a complete holistic system for the reduction of suffering. The most complete expression of this *Darśana* is the *Yoga Sūtras of* Patañjali, compiled in the first century BCE.

Little is known about the historical facts of Patañjali's life. Nonetheless, this great sage is highly esteemed, not only for his contributions to *Yoga*, but for authoring foundational texts on

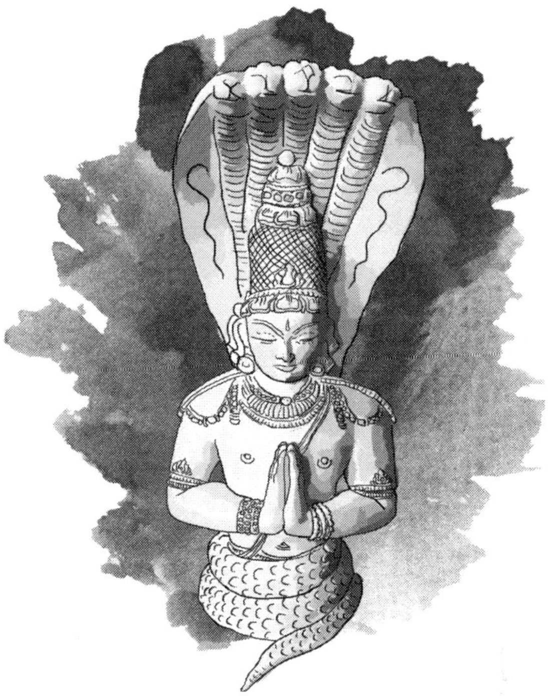

Patanjali

Sanskrit grammar and *Āyurveda* (a system of traditional Indian medicine). The *Yoga Sūtras* were compiled by this great sage over 2,300 years ago. A testament to their enduring value is that these profound teachings are still studied, chanted and practiced by *Yoga* devotees worldwide as a means of reducing suffering.

A *sūtra* is a form of writing characterized by short phrases or aphorisms with a depth of meaning. These teachings require a qualified teacher to help interpret and apply them to our lives. The *Yoga Sūtras* are universal and do not profess any one belief system. In the *sūtras*, we find many of the ideas introduced in the *Vedas* and clarified in the *Upaniṣads* and *Bhagavad Gītā* compiled in a single text. The 195 *sūtras* contained in the four chapters of the *Yoga Sūtras* present the essence of *Yoga*.

Chapter I introduces *Yoga*, its meaning, purpose and goal: to cultivate a mind that is able to choose and focus on an object despite distractions. The object we choose must be in alignment with our goal. In this chapter, Patañjali presents the tools for achieving this quality of mind, describes the obstacles we might encounter and offers suggestions for overcoming them.

Chapter II outlines the fundamental source of human suffering (the *Kleśas*), the formula for relieving that suffering (*Kriyā Yoga*) and the tools (*Aṣṭāṅga Yoga*) for sustainable change.

Chapter III outlines the powers available to one who has mastered the art of meditation. Patañjali lists possible objects of focus in meditation and their various benefits, while cautioning us as to the potential misuse of powers gained from meditation.

Chapter IV is aimed at the most advanced student of *Yoga*. It states that the path to lasting freedom (*kaivalya*) lies in realizing the subtle but essential distinction between spirit and matter. It also clarifies that the role of the teacher is to support the student in this realization.

The *Yoga Sūtras* and Religion

In the *Yoga Sūtras*, there are several significant distinctions between *Yoga* and religion:

In religion, the belief in God is primary, essential and non-negotiable. In Patañjali's *Yoga Sūtras*, a relationship with God is optional.

In religion, some variation of union with God is the goal. In *Yoga*, union with God is offered as a possible tool to achieve *Yoga*'s goals of clarity of mind and freedom from mental suffering.

In the various world religions, the role of God is seen as the great father figure or an all-powerful creator, sustainer and destroyer to whom we must surrender our power. In the *sūtras*, God is described as the first teacher, the self-empowering source from which all teachings flow.

Throughout its history, *Yoga* has continued to evolve to accommodate the changing needs and challenges of the people and the times. This living tradition can be a state of mind, a practice, a philosophy or a way of life. As you make your way through this book, we invite you to reflect on what *Yoga* is and what it can be for you.

To Sum Up:

- Modern *Yoga* is a system whose roots date back to the ancient Indian *Vedic* teaching.
- *Yoga* is not a religion, though it helps to deepen one's spiritual beliefs.
- *Yoga* is one of the six *Darśanas*, India's classical philosophies for reducing human suffering.
- Based on *Sāṃkhya Darśana*, suffering is reduced by creating a more sattvic mind.
- Patañjali's *Yoga Sūtras* is the source text for the *Darśana* of *Yoga*.

CHAPTER 2

The *Yoga* of T. Krishnamacharya

Throughout its history, *Yoga* has continued to evolve and expand to suit the ever-changing needs of humanity. One of the most influential and innovative *Yoga* teachers of modern times was a South Indian named Śrī Tirumalai Krishnamacharya (1888-1989), a *Vedic* scholar and healer who held advanced degrees in philosophy, *Āyurveda*, Sanskrit and music. This enigmatic teacher, who was known simply as T. Krishnamacharya, was both a classicist who revered the ancient traditions and a fearless innovator willing to minimize or disregard any teachings he felt were no longer relevant to the times.

This *Yoga* master was firmly rooted in the traditional lineage model of *Yoga* in which, much like the *Vedas*, the teachings were handed down from teacher to student to preserve their integrity. T. Krishnamacharya taught what he learned from his teacher to his student and son T.K.V. Desikachar (1938-2016), who in turn taught our teachers. Now, we are passing them on to you. Anytime we use the word "lineage" in this book we are referring to these teachers and the specific teachings that have been handed down.

Although T. Krishnamacharya was a devout Hindu, he emphasized the universality of *Yoga* and brought three dramatic innovations to this ancient healing art:

Gender accessibility

He taught *Yoga* to women at a time when it was still a strict discipline into which only young boys were admitted. Furthermore, he predicted that it would be women who would play a key role in carrying *Yoga* into the future. An examination of the disproportionate ratio of women to men in today's *Yoga* classes confirms his prediction.

Individualization

In T. Krishnamacharya's effort to make *Yoga* more available to a wider spectrum of people, he developed modifications and adaptations of its many tools. This made the practice of *Yoga* more suitable to each student's unique needs, strengths, limitations and goals.

Secularization of *Yoga*

For centuries, the vast majority of *Yoga* practitioners were Hindus. By separating the tightly woven strands of *Yoga* and Hinduism, T. Krishnamacharya made *Yoga* more relevant to the masses, regardless of their religious beliefs. His approach emphasized *Yoga*'s universality, while diminishing any religious associations.

Styles and Approaches

In modern times, we have witnessed the emergence of numerous styles of *Yoga* practice. In these approaches, the student, regardless of his or her age, must adhere to the specific guidelines and characteristics of that style.

Rather than styles, T. Krishnamacharya offered five distinct methodologies of *Yoga* practices: *Sṛṣṭi Krama, Śikṣaṇa Krama, Rakṣaṇa Krama, Ādhyātmika Krama* and *Cikitsā Krama*, each of which is tailored to the individual. These classical approaches correspond to the three stages of life (student, householder and sunset) found in both the *Vedas* and in *Āyurveda* (traditional Indian medicine). They are as relevant today as they were millennia ago.

The Three Stages of Life

Based on *Vedic* teachings, T. Krishnamacharya recognized that life was divided into three distinct stages. In the **student stage**, defined as childhood to the early 20s, the aim is cultivating the discipline needed for rigorous study, increased stamina and physical development. To achieve this, the practices are long and strenuous, with a primary focus on more athletic *āsana* (physical postures).

Next is the **householder stage**, approximately 25 to 65 years of age. Here the purpose of practice is to provide the stability needed during midlife to maintain good health and support the responsibilities incumbent upon an active adult. During this stage the practice periods are shorter to accommodate the busy lifestyle of a householder. The *āsana* is less athletic, with greater emphasis on breath control. It takes into account the age, occupation, health needs and other factors specific to the individual. To help improve mental focus, clarify values and enrich the life of the practitioner, *prāṇāyāma* (control and regulation of the breath) and meditation were also integrated into the practice.

The **sunset stage** begins when the practitioner is freed from the daily responsibilities of working and raising a family. Here the practice is far more contemplative, with just enough movement to keep the body flexible, the mind attentive and maintain vitality. As the goal at this stage is to enable the elder to ponder life's mysteries and meaning, the emphasis is on *prāṇāyāma*, meditation, reflection and ritual.

The Five *Kramas*

Krishnamacharya developed and taught five different methodologies (*Kramas*) based on the *Vedic* stage-of-life model, as well as on his extensive knowledge of *Āyurveda* and the *Yoga Sūtras*. The practices he designed within each *Krama* were highly individualized, taking into account each person's constitution, health needs, lifestyle and personal goals.

In ***Sṛṣṭi Krama*** the emphasis is on developing strength, flexibility, confidence and discipline. Designed for children, this *Krama* includes both moving and static postures in preparation for more challenging *vinyāsas* (series of poses linked together). To intensify this practice, the recitation of sounds, chants or *mantras* are used to help lengthen the breath and focus the mind.

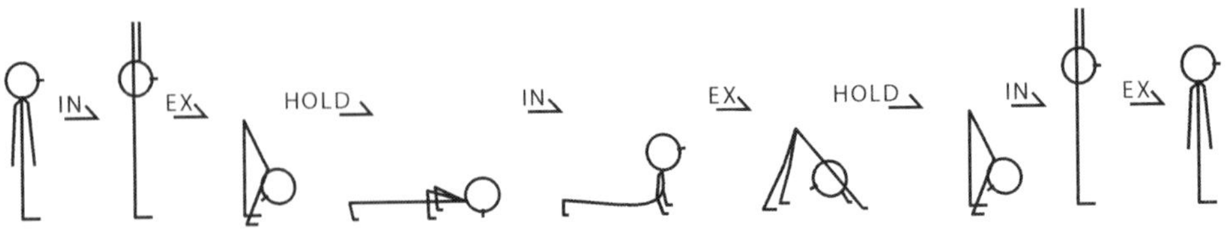

Sṛṣṭi Krama vinyāsa

Śikṣaṇa Krama emphasizes mastery of the classical postures and introduces conscious breathing. Originally aimed at young adults, this approach strives for perfection in posture and breath. The goal of this *Krama* is to develop the physical stamina and mental focus needed for meditation. The *Śikṣaṇa* approach is appropriate for anyone with the ability, motivation and time required to accomplish this mastery.

Rakṣaṇa Krama practices are designed to maintain optimal health, protect the physical body and prevent injury and disease. Aimed at the householder, a greater range of *Yoga's* tools (*āsana, prāṇāyāma,* meditation, chanting, ritual and study) are combined and adapted to the individual's needs in order to sustain mental and physical stability. With mastery of postures no longer a concern, these rich practices are shorter in duration to allow practitioners the time needed for their jobs, family and societal duties.

Ādhyātmika Krama consists of more contemplative practices that emphasize meditation, prayer and ritual to achieve inner peace and self-realization. These practices are taught to individuals free from the demands of daily living, typically those in the later stages of life. This approach enables them to focus on deeper spiritual or religious practices for which they previously lacked the time due to the demands of daily living.

Cikitsā Krama is *Yoga* therapy and can be implemented at any stage of life. It uses tools and practices based on classic healing models such as *Āyurveda* to address and manage specific health issues. For this purpose, *Cikitsā* modifies and integrates the tools of *āsana, prāṇāyāma,* meditation, visualization, sound, ritual and prayer found in the other *Kramas*. It also utilizes the *Āyurvedic* tools of diet, herbs, massage and lifestyle modification. Today, *Cikitsā Krama* is seen more as a complement to Western medicine than as a replacement for regular checkups and professional medical care.

In keeping with his respect for individualization, T. Krishnamacharya taught that components of all five classical approaches can be combined and practiced at any stage of life, provided they are based on the specific needs of the practitioner.

T. Krishnamacharya's Definitions of *Yoga*

Based on his extensive knowledge of the *Veda*s and the *Amarakośa* (an ancient Sanskrit thesaurus), T. Krishnamacharya offered five definitions of *Yoga*. These definitions link the practice of this ancient healing art with both universal principles and the demands of everyday living:

- ***Sannāha*** is the preparation taken before beginning a journey toward a goal.
- ***Upāya*** is the ability to do something tomorrow that was not possible today.
- ***Saṁgati*** means to link two objects together.
- ***Dhyāna*** is continuous focused attention.
- ***Yukti*** is the skillful use of appropriate tools or strategies to achieve a desired result.

To Sum Up:

- T. Krishnamacharya was a highly influential *Yoga* teacher who was both a classicist and an innovator.
- T. Krishnamacharya developed three dramatic innovations to *Yoga*:
  1. He taught *Yoga* to women.
  2. He individualized *Yoga* practices.
  3. He separated *Yoga* and religion.
- The ancient *Vedas* describe three stages of life:
  1. student
  2. householder
  3. sunset
- T. Krishnamacharya's teachings are based on five functional approaches:
  1. *Sṛṣṭi Krama* emphasizes discipline and development.
  2. *Śikṣaṇa Krama* is aimed at perfection and mastery.
  3. *Rakṣaṇa Krama* addresses prevention and maintenance.
  4. *Ādhyātmika Krama* promotes reflection and spirituality.
  5. *Cikitsā Krama* focuses on therapeutic applications.
- T. Krishnamacharya offered five definitions of *Yoga*:
  1. preparatory steps taken before beginning a journey toward a goal
  2. the ability to do something tomorrow that was not possible today
  3. linking two objects together
  4. continuous focused attention
  5. skillful use of the appropriate tools or strategies to achieve a desired result

CHAPTER 3

The Underlying Causes of Human Suffering: The Five *Kleśas*

According to Patañjali, there are five inherent tendencies in the mind that are the source of all human suffering. Collectively, they are known as the *kleśas* (afflictions): misperceiving reality, confusing our self-image, excessive craving, unreasonable avoidance and the many forms of fear. It is essential to have a basic understanding of these ***kleśas*** and how they distort our perceptions, choices and behaviors.

One important distinction: though these tendencies don't always lead to suffering, whenever there is suffering, the *kleśas* are always the cause.

Misperceiving reality, or ***avidyā***, is the root *kleśa* underlying the other four. Have you ever gone on a spending spree in denial that you are deeply in debt? Do you find yourself trying to gain approval from someone (a boss, a boyfriend or a *Yoga* teacher) in order to feel good about yourself only to find it doesn't work? The ensuing discomfort in both cases is the result of our misperception. *Yoga* teaches that the ultimate misperception of reality, the deepest *avidyā*, is confusing our unchanging spirit (*puruṣa*) with the ever-changing material world (*prakṛti*).

Confused self-image, ***asmitā***, causes us to identify our true value with things inside or outside of ourselves, all of which are subject to change. When we base our self-worth solely on things such as our car, profession or the shape of our body, it will always lead to suffering.

Excessive craving, ***rāga***, is the next *kleśa*. This affliction causes us to pursue something which once brought us pleasure, despite negative consequences. Are you the runner who craves the surge of endorphins from your daily run, even though you experience pain in your knees? Do you know a gambler or drinker who keeps chasing the initial high, even though their life is falling apart? Though *rāga* in the extreme is addiction, we have all experienced wanting something even though we know we will regret it later.

The next *kleśa* is aversion, ***dveṣa***. Here, the expectation of pain causes us to avoid something even though it may no longer be a problem. If you've ever gotten food poisoning from a restaurant, you've probably never returned. Later, when your best friend's engagement party is planned at the restaurant, you refuse to go. Even though the restaurant is now under new ownership, the aversion you feel is so strong you are willing to hurt your friend's feelings rather than revisit the scene of your bad experience. This level of aversion will always lead to suffering.

Fear that prevents us from living a rich, full life is ***abhiniveśa***. Ultimately, it is the fear of dying. Do you avoid flying because of your fear of heights or enclosed spaces? Have you ever broken out in a cold sweat when you have to speak in front of a crowd? According to the *sūtras, abhiniveśa* is a powerful emotion with its own momentum from which no one is immune.

One undeniable fact is that life is always changing. The mind's resistance to change is the fertile soil in which the *kleśas* take root. By understanding the various stages of the *kleśas* we can prevent their negative effects.

The Stages of the *Kleśas*

The ***kleśas*** exist in three progressive stages: dormant, rising and full blown. According to the *sutras*, by taking preventative steps to control them while they are in their earlier, less intense stages, we minimize their negative effects.

Here is an example of the complete cycle of *rāga* (craving). Janet tends to over-indulge in sweets, so she would be wise to maintain a sugar-free house and avoid bakeries. She goes out to dinner with friends with no intention of having dessert (dormant). As the dessert tray rolls by, her craving for sweets rises to the surface and she is tempted to indulge (rising). At this point, Janet still has a choice whether to maintain self-control or give in to her cravings. Her friend orders chocolate cake and offers her a taste. Thinking that this will be a good compromise, she accepts it. When Janet puts the first bite of luscious chocolate cake in her mouth, her tendency to over-indulge kicks in and she has little to no chance of stopping and orders her own. Now the *rāga* is full-blown.

This example shows why it is important to learn to recognize the *kleśas* in their early stages and take preventative measures. Had she been proactive by asking her friend, beforehand, if she were going to have dessert, Janet could have caught her *rāga* before it started to rise. By the time the dessert had arrived, her *rāga* was full-blown and she was unable to make a conscious choice.

Often, one *kleśa* is stronger and will dominate the other. For instance, even though Janet believes that fitting into a smaller dress size would bring her lasting happiness (*asmitā*), this belief was outweighed by the craving for the dessert (*rāga)* that led to her eating a piece of cake.

A *kleśa* reflection: Which *kleśa* affects you the most? How has it caused you to suffer? What preventative measures can you take to address this *kleśa* while in its dormant state? When, in your experience, has one *kleśa* dominated over another?

To Sum Up:

- The source of all suffering is the five inherent mental tendencies known as the *kleśas*:
  1. *avidyā* — misperceiving reality
  2. *asmitā* — confused self-image
  3. *rāga* — excessive craving
  4. *dveṣa* — unreasonable aversion
  5. *abhiniveśa* — fear of ending, the unknown and ultimately death
- The *kleśas* can be dormant, rising or full-blown.
- We should take preventative actions when the *kleśas* are dormant.
- One *kleśa* can override another.

CHAPTER 4

The Yoga of Action: *Kriyā Yoga*

According to the *sūtras*, we suffer because our minds cling to the familiar and to what once worked, even though our lives are constantly changing. Recognizing both the need for change and the mind's resistance to it, the *Yoga Sūtras* of Patañjali offers the ***Kriyā Yoga* Model**, "the *Yoga* of action." This model presents three interrelated components which, when combined, present a clear path for changing habits and creating sustainable transformation.

The first component in *Kriyā Yoga* is ***tapas***: initiating new, often challenging, behaviors needed to create positive changes in our lives. Commonly, it is the awareness of our own suffering that provides the impetus needed to change these behaviors. Sickness motivates us to refine our diet. The desire for a higher paying job encourages us to develop new skills or complete a training program. Whatever the cause, adopting new behaviors, *tapas*, is an essential element in *Kriyā Yoga*.

The second component of *Kriyā Yoga* is ***svādhyāya***, or self-reflection. Such introspection guides us in choosing the correct *tapas*. This self-observation continues during the performance of the *tapas*. Once we've taken the appropriate action, further reflection helps verify that we've made the right choice. For example, because our excess weight is causing high blood pressure, we decide to change our diet. After weeks of eating differently, we notice that we have shed some pounds and our blood pressure has gone down. This confirms we have chosen the right *tapas*.

Today, we use coaches, therapists and spiritual advisors to guide us in our reflection. In the *Yoga* model, however, the most reliable references have always been teachers with whom we have a heart to heart relationship.

The third component is *īśvarapraṇidhāna*, the ability to focus on the quality of our actions rather than on the outcome. This concept has many interpretations, but when it is present in our actions, there is trust, teachability and a willingness to change. Because *Kriyā Yoga* is a step into the unknown, *īśvarapraṇidhāna* is an indispensable factor.

Here is an example that illustrates these concepts in everyday life.

Fran's story:

"For years, I had a vision of owning a *Yoga* studio to teach and offer classes in a calm, comfortable environment. After much hard work, my dream became a reality. For many years, I experienced great joy and contentment teaching in the space I had created.

Gradually, though, the day-to-day stresses of running a business began to outweigh the enjoyment I received from teaching. Soon, I saw the need for some kind of change but found that this was easier said than done. For two long years, I experienced an increasing dissatisfaction with the daily affairs of running a business. It was only after several enlightening conversations with my mentor, and much reflection, that something clicked. I realized that my identity as a *Yoga* teacher had become confused with that of a studio owner. I explored various options for changing my situation and eventually let my studio go and returned to my true love, teaching *Yoga*."

Fran succeeded in creating a dramatic transformation through *Kriyā Yoga*. Closing the studio was her *tapas*. Although difficult, letting go of the studio was precisely the action needed to reduce her suffering and improve the quality of her life.

Her *svādhyāya*, with the help of her teacher, was essential in choosing the correct *tapas*. Later, reflection on her increased enthusiasm for teaching confirmed that she made the right move. Finally, her willingness to follow her teacher's advice and let go of the past, with no expectation of future results, was a measure of Fran's *īśvarapraṇidhāna*.

Kriyā Yoga begins with the awareness that we are suffering and a belief that change is possible. As the above story illustrates, the three components of *Kriyā Yoga* could occur in any order. It might begin with self-reflection (*svādhyāya)* to help clarify our goals and develop a strategy of action. Sometimes, we start by taking an action (*tapas)* in an attempt to alleviate our suffering and reflect on it later. Other times, we are so overwhelmed that we reach out to someone or something beyond ourselves in which we have faith (*īśvarapraṇidhāna*) for guidance. However we begin, *Kriyā Yoga* is an ongoing practice which creates positive change and continual improvement in our lives.

To Sum Up:

- We have a tendency to hold on to habits that produce predictable results, even though they no longer serve us. Patañjali's three-part *Kriyā Yoga* Model provides a solution to this problem.
- There are three components of *Kriyā Yoga*:

  1. initiating new behaviors, *tapas*
  2. personal observation and reflection, *svādhyāya*
  3. focusing on the quality of our actions rather than on the outcome, *īśvarapraṇidhāna*

CHAPTER 5

The Eight Limbs/*Aṣṭāṅga Yoga*: Tools for Transformation

All four chapters of the *Yoga Sūtras* are rich with insights and strategies to facilitate personal growth and positive change in our lives. In the second chapter, Patañjali presents the most powerful, concrete and specific tools for transformation, known as *Aṣṭāṅga Yoga*, or the eight limbs. This holistic model offers guidelines for balanced (*sattvic*) living in the areas of relationships, lifestyle, body, breath, senses and the mind.

The eight limbs are *yamas, niyamas, āsana, prāṇāyāma, pratyāhāra, dhāraṇā, dhyāna* and *samādhi*. This chapter offers a brief introduction to these limbs; there will be a more in-depth exploration in the chapters that follow.

Yamas

The first limb, *yamas*, can be thought of as "relationship guidelines." These recommendations address our behaviors and attitudes with respect to other people and the world. Specifically, the *yamas* give us advice for cultivating kinder, more honest interpersonal relationships and suggestions for living in harmony with our natural environment.

Niyamas

The *niyamas*, the second limb, refers to our personal lifestyle, as well as the attitudes and behaviors we maintain with respect to ourselves. The *niyamas* encourage us to develop healthier habits in every area of our daily lives.

Āsana

Āsana, the third limb in Patanjali's model, refers to the physical postures. While it is impossible to stretch your way to sustained joy, when *āsana* is performed with stability and comfort in equal measure, the result is improved physical, mental and emotional well-being.

Prāṇāyāma

The fourth limb, *prāṇāyāma*, is a set of guidelines for control and regulation of the breath. This powerful practice improves all physiological functions and is essential in cultivating a more stable mind. Ultimately, the goal of *prāṇāyāma* is to develop a long, smooth breath and prepare the mind for meditation.

Pratyāhāra

Pratyāhāra, the fifth limb, explains that, when used properly, the senses are simply an instrument of our consciousness. Through *pratyāhāra*, the senses allow us to appreciate the external world, while not distracting us from the internal.

Dhāraṇā

Dhāraṇā, the sixth limb, is the first step in the process of meditation. This step requires the ability to choose an object of interest upon which we can direct our attention. Focusing on the appropriate object helps to steady the mind as well as enrich and improve our lives.

Dhyāna

In *dhyāna*, the seventh limb, the mind continues its focus on and develops a strong connection with the chosen object. As a result, we learn more about both the qualities of the chosen object and ourselves. Though meditation is, in fact, a multistage process, *dhyāna* is the one word considered synonymous with meditation.

Samādhi

In the eighth limb, *samādhi*, the meditator becomes completely absorbed in the object of meditation. In this state of focused attention, we become so completely absorbed in the object that we lose all sense of self. In *samādhi*, we are free from the normal mental activities that distract and define us.

Whether we are treating ourselves or others with more respect, learning to control our body and breath, or meditating on a chosen object, the key to transformation lies in consistent practice of the eight limbs.

To Sum Up:

- The second chapter of the *Yoga Sūtras* contains the most potent tools for transformation.
- The tools are presented in the form of a holistic model called the eight limbs or *Aṣṭāṅga Yoga*.
- This model offers guidelines for balanced living.
- The eight limbs are:

  1. *yama* — relationships
  2. *niyama* — lifestyle
  3. *āsana* — body
  4. *prāṇāyāma* — breath
  5. *pratyāhāra* — controlling the senses
  6. *dhāraṇā* — concentration
  7. *dhyāna* — meditation
  8. *samādhi* — absorption

CHAPTER 6

The First Limb/*Yamas*: Principles for Positive Relationships

"The true test of whether or not our *Yoga* is working is that our relationships improve."

T.K.V. Desikachar

We are always in relationship. From the moment we're born, our health, well-being and very existence are rooted in our connection to other people and the environment. The five *yamas* are foundational principles for cultivating more-respectful, more-conscious relationships with everyone and everything around us. They are *ahiṁsā* (kindness), *satya* (truthfulness), *asteya* (honesty), *brahmacharya* (moderation) and *aparigraha* (enoughness).

Rather than advocating rigid adherence to a traditional system of right and wrong or good and bad, the *yamas* encourage us to increase awareness of our behaviors and their consequences. To fully understand the deeper significance of the *yamas*, one must go beyond morals, ethics and religious dogma.

We all know how challenging relationships can be. In fact, sometimes they seem like an impossible balancing act. It's a constant struggle to be honest with ourselves without hurting other's feelings, and it's equally hard to be kind to others while being true to ourselves. Because we usually feel like we give more than we receive in any given relationship, we often end up feeling like we're being treated unfairly. In addition, when we fail to see the interconnectedness between ourselves and nature, we inadvertently exploit and abuse our environment at the cost of our own health and well-being.

How do we resolve this seemingly inevitable predicament? Patañjali offers five guidelines for improving our relationships with people and our environment.

Ahiṁsā

Ahiṁsā, translated as respect for life and kindness for all living things, is the root principle upon which the other four *yamas* are based.

To get to the heart of *ahiṁsā*, we need to look at how we treat others, as well as the underlying attitudes behind these behaviors. We are often unaware of, or in denial about, how our attitudes and actions (or failure to act) negatively impact others. The *yamas* teach us to be more conscious of our interactions in the world and help us cultivate more positive and proactive behaviors. As with every other practice in *Yoga*, the *yamas* both require and lead to self-reflection (*svādhyāya*). Observing that I've deliberately or unconsciously insulted my partner, friend or neighbor, for example, provides me with an opportunity to reflect on any anger, negativity and resentment I've been holding inside. Noticing that I have caused harm to another enables me to reflect on the source of these actions and take the necessary steps to create more-respectful behavior, or *ahiṁsā*. This same principle can be applied to our relationship with the environment. For example, we should make a greater effort to reduce our carbon footprint with the looming threat of climate change.

Suggestions for practicing *ahiṁsā*:

- Praise a friend or family member the next time we see them.
- Accept responsibility and apologize when we have said or done something that has hurt another's feelings, even if it was unintentional.
- Practice listening to others more intently by letting them finish their sentences and by waiting a moment before we respond.
- Respect the environment by conserving energy and recycling.

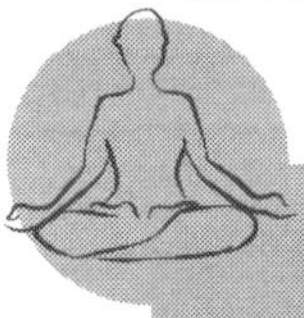

Ahiṁsā Practice:

- Find a comfortable, seated position.
- Take 10 breaths.
- On inhale, mentally recite "May kindness fill my heart."
- On exhale, recite "Let this kindness extend to all beings."
- Sit quietly and set the intention for kindness to guide your day.
- Practice this regularly and reflect on the results.

Satya

The second *yama*, *satya*, is defined as telling the truth or being honest in our communication. Building on the principle of *ahiṁsā*, we work on telling the truth in a way that it can be heard and does not cause harm. This is beautifully expressed by T.K.V. Desikachar, "Tell the truth that is pleasant, don't tell the truth that is unpleasant, and don't lie just because it is pleasant."

Suggestions for practicing *satya*:

- Before we say something, reflect on whether this is the best possible time. If we are tired, hungry or distracted, it will probably be reflected in our tone and might not be heard the way it was intended
- Make an effort to communicate clearly, in a way that will not cause harm. This prevents us from needing to make amends in the future.
- Always consider the person we are talking to. Some people are more sensitive than others.

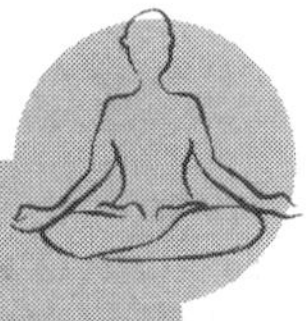

Satya Practice:

- Find a comfortable, seated position.
- Take 10 breaths.
- On inhale, mentally recite "Give me clarity to know the truth."
- On exhale, recite "Let that truth be expressed in my communications."
- Sit quietly and set the intention to let truthfulness guide your day.
- Practice this regularly and reflect on the results.

Asteya

While *satya* refers to being honest in our communication, *asteya* (not stealing), requires that we apply the same honesty in all our actions. This includes not taking property, time, information or anything else that does not belong to us or which has not been given freely. Though this obviously refers to shoplifting or stealing a car, it also includes less-obvious, everyday offenses such as cheating on taxes, "borrowing" office supplies from a place of employment and showing up late (stealing another person's time). Though these activities are often perceived as acceptable behavior and not theft, the goal of *Yoga* is to bring more consciousness to our rationalizations on stealing, its effects on society and on our own psyches.

Suggestions for practicing *asteya*:

- Work on cultivating a feeling of already having enough. If we believe there is more than enough to go around, stealing isn't necessary.
- Reflect on our own definition of acceptable theft and any rationalizations that support it.

Asteya Practice:

- Find a comfortable, seated position.
- Take 10 breaths.
- On inhale, mentally recite "I have all that I need to thrive."
- On exhale, recite "I share whenever I'm able."
- Sit quietly and envision that you're surrounded by abundance.
- Practice this regularly and reflect on the results.

Brahmacharya

Though *brahmacharya* is commonly understood as celibacy, a more accurate definition is practicing moderation and not allowing distractions to get in the way of achieving our highest goals. For a college student with the goal of earning a degree, *brahmacharya* behavior would be eating well, limiting the partying and getting enough sleep. This kind of moderation will provide the student with the needed time and energy to pursue their studies and accomplish their goals. If we have a career and are responsible for a family, *brahmacharya* behavior would include practicing monogamy, living within our means and conserving our energy for our home life and job.

Suggestions for practicing *brahmacharya:*

- Reflect regularly on our priorities and goals.
- Before acting impulsively, consider how our behavior will impact our current life situation.
- Examine our choices to ensure that they help fulfill our daily responsibilities.

Brahmacharya Practice:

- Find a comfortable, seated position.
- Take 10 breaths.
- On inhale, mentally recite "I am clear about my goals."
- On exhale, recite "I am directing my energy to achieving them."
- Sit quietly and set the intention that you are committed to a course that will lead to the accomplishment of your goal.
- Practice this regularly and reflect on the results.

Aparigraha

As the saying goes, "At some point, we merely become caretakers to the things we own." The final *yama, aparigraha* (not grasping) is about cultivating the feeling of having enough and reducing our endless desire for more. This attitude applies to things, experiences, knowledge, relationships and many other possessions. We live in a consumer-based society where we are constantly bombarded by messages, both overtly and subliminally, that we don't have enough. The purpose of *aparigraha* is to increase our sense of satisfaction by clarifying which objects are essential for our comfort and security and which are unnecessary and burdensome.

With regular *Yoga* practice, we gain increased discernment and serenity by learning what frees us from *aparigraha*'s self-perpetuating grasp.

Suggestions for practicing *aparigraha*:

- Clean out your closet and donate any unused possessions. Anything you haven't touched in one year is probably dispensable.
- Reduce impulse buying by waiting 24 hours, giving yourself time to reflect on whether it truly contributes to your life.
- Regularly express gratitude for everything you have. This will help cultivate a feeling of abundance.

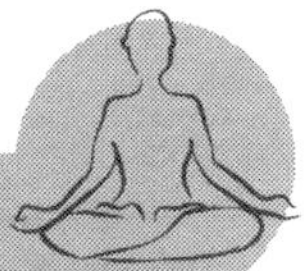

Aparigraha Practice:

- Find a comfortable, seated position.
- Take 10 breaths.
- On inhale, mentally recite "I am grateful for all that I have."
- On exhale, recite "I have everything that I need."
- Set the intention that you already have all you need to be happy.
- Practice this regularly and reflect on the results.

The *yamas* support us in relating to people and the environment with integrity, respect and a sense of wholeness. They are both the first step on the *Yoga* path and, ultimately, the measure of how well *Yoga* is working in our lives.

To Sum Up:

- The *yamas* are principles for cultivating more-conscious relationships.
- The five *yamas* are:
  1. *ahiṁsā* — respect and kindness
  2. *satya* — truthfulness
  3. *asteya* — honesty
  4. *brahmacharya* — moderation
  5. *aparigraha* — enoughness
- The *yamas* support us in relating to people and the environment with integrity, respect and a sense of wholeness.
- The *yamas* are both the first step on the *Yoga* path and, ultimately, the measure of how well *Yoga* is working in our lives.

CHAPTER 7

The Second Limb/*Niyamas*: Guidelines for a Balanced Lifestyle

Yoga's second limb, the *niyamas*, is a set of guidelines to help us cultivate discipline and overcome our innate resistance to change. This begins with reflecting on the relationship between our beliefs and attitudes and how they affect our behaviors. The five *niyamas* encourage us to develop healthier habits in every aspect of our daily lives. They are *śauca* (cleanliness), *saṁtoṣa* (contentment), *tapas* (new behavior), *svādhyāya* (reflection) and *īśvarapraṇidhāna* (acceptance).

We all tend to develop habits and cling to them even when they cause suffering. Clearly, we need to change, but excessive desire, lack of discipline and fear of the unknown often sabotage our best attempts. Patañjali, in his wisdom, addresses the difficulty of changing our behaviors by offering a simple progression of steps for transformation, beginning with the body.

Śauca

Just as regular maintenance of our car is required for it to run well, we must give the same quality of care to our physical body and state of mind. The first *niyama, śauca* (cleanliness or purity) encourages proper physical hygiene, appropriate food choices, good personal grooming and maintenance of our physical well-being. In addition, it refers to living our lives with a sense of order and organization, which includes keeping our environment neat and clean and our affairs in order.

Yoga teaches that, while the physical body can be seen as merely a container for our consciousness, it is nonetheless a precious gift that needs to be respected and maintained.

Suggestions for practicing *śauca*:

- Observe daily personal hygiene. This could include bathing, skin brushing, tongue scraping, etc.
- Exercise regularly and eat whole, healthy foods to nourish the body.
- Practice seasonal guided fasting or cleansing aimed at detoxification.
- Treat yourself to bodywork such as massage and acupressure to help reduce toxins.
- Seek out the support needed to maintain sound mental and emotional health.

Saṁtoṣa

Saṁtoṣa, the second *niyama*, is translated as contentment. Developing the ability to be happy with what we have leads to feelings of peace and harmony. In a consumer culture where we tend to believe that more is better and that happiness can be bought, we are continuously inundated with the message that what we have and who we are is never quite enough. *Saṁtoṣa* is the realization that, ultimately, contentment comes, not from things outside ourselves, but from within.

To practice *saṁtoṣa*, we strive to cultivate an attitude of gratitude, refrain from social comparison and establish a feeling of enoughness. This principle is the antidote to greed and entitlement, encouraging us to be satisfied with who we are and what we already have. *Saṁtoṣa* is the ability to appreciate all the riches the world has to offer without needing to own them.

Suggestions for practicing *saṁtoṣa*:

- Acknowledge others' good fortunes without feeling envy.
- Create a daily list of things we are grateful for.
- Give to others who are less fortunate.
- Be aware of the powerful influence of the endless stream of advertising.

Tapas

Tapas is a term first presented in the *Kriyā Yoga* model. As a *niyama*, it means to change personal behaviors that no longer serve us. Practicing *tapas*, though not always easy, shines a light on our unconscious behaviors and helps to create new habits. For some, practicing *tapas* means getting more exercise, while for others it might be less activity and more rest. For certain individuals, it may entail eating more vegetables, while others need to give up sugar and caffeine. Although changing our behavior is initially challenging, it eventually becomes easier and provides insights on how our habits are formed.

Suggestions for practicing *tapas*:

- Replace sedentary behavior with an appropriate *āsana* practice, walking or other exercise to help strengthen and purify the physical body.
- Eliminate foods that were once easily digestible but now aggravate your system.
- Replace unhealthy comfort foods with those that are more nutritional.
- Reduce habitual activities that over-stimulate the senses, such as spending too much time on the internet, watching television or playing video games.
- Encourage mental alertness by engaging in educational activities, such as learning a new language, art or skill.

Svādhyāya

Svādhyāya is the ability to observe and reflect on one's own actions and accurately assess their consequences. *Svādhyāya*, when practiced with the support of a teacher, mentor or wisdom text, provides us with fresh insights, alternative viewpoints and increased self-awareness. Our progress in *Yoga* depends on the quality of such observations and reflections, as well as our willingness to take actions based on them.

Suggestions for practicing *svādhyāya*:

- Examine self-limiting beliefs, habitual attitudes and patterns of behaviors.
- Keep a journal on things that inspire you or significant events of the day.
- Write down your long and short-term goals.
- Verify your reflections with a trusted teacher, mentor, therapist or guide.

Īśvarapraṇidhāna

Īśvarapraṇidhāna is another term from the *Kriyā Yoga* model. Here, it encourages us to focus on the quality of our day-to-day activities, rather than their results. *Īśvarapraṇidhāna* also refers to having the courage and humility to accept the fact that there are always forces beyond our control.

This guiding principle encourages us to remain open and teachable in all our affairs. Finally, a strong sense of *īśvarapraṇidhāna* gives us the confidence to venture into the unknown territory of new behavior.

Suggestions for practicing *īśvarapraṇidhāna*:

- Have the courage to try something new every day.
- Cultivate the faith that in the end everything will work out.
- Recite the first stanza of Reinhold Niebuhr's famous "Serenity Prayer" and reflect on its meaning:

  God grant me the serenity to accept the things I cannot change;

  The courage to change the things I can;

  And the wisdom to know the difference.

To Sum Up:

- The *niyamas* are guidelines for cultivating a more conscious lifestyle.
- Practicing the *niyamas* helps to create personal transformation by encouraging us to make more refined choices in our daily life.
- The *niyamas* are:

  1. *śauca* — cleanliness
  2. *saṁtoṣa* — contentment
  3. *tapas* — new behaviors
  4. *svādhyāya* — reflection
  5. *īśvarapraṇidhāna* — acceptance

CHAPTER 8

The Third Limb/*Āsana*: Moving the body

As far back as 3,000 BCE, cave dwellers decorated their walls with drawings of people in *Yoga āsana*. Since that time, volumes have been written about the source and evolution of these postures. Although *āsana* is only one of *Yoga*'s many tools, it has become the most popular and recognizable. Let's take a brief look at *āsana's* possible origins. Though none of these explanations can be positively verified, the following three mythological stories have resonated most deeply throughout the ages.

Myth One

Ancient sages, the first *yogis*, studied the forms and behaviors of various animals and objects in nature. They believed it was possible to gain the poise of a cobra, the vision of an eagle and the flexible strength of a tree by mimicking these natural shapes.

Myth Two

Ancient *ṛṣis* (wise men) became filled with powerful energy while practicing meditation. This caused them to move spontaneously, bending their bodies into various shapes and poses. Later, having returned to their normal state of mind, they deliberately tried to recreate these poses (which became *āsana*) in the hope that, by doing so, they could enter into the same states of ecstasy they had experienced while meditating.

Myth Three

In this story, *Vedic* astrologers inform a couple that their newborn son, Matsyendra, was born under unlucky stars. Upon hearing this, his parents throw him into the ocean, where he is promptly swallowed by a giant fish whose belly becomes his new home. At the same time, in another part of the universe, Śiva, the great Hindu God, agrees to teach his partner, Parvati, the secrets of *Yoga*. To ensure privacy, he transports them to the bottom of the ocean, where he reveals the secret teachings. In the middle of the lesson, the giant fish, with the young Matsyendra still in his belly, comes swimming by, allowing the boy to hear the teachings. He becomes a student of *Yoga*, practicing *āsana* for twelve years, while still living in the belly of the fish. Later, as a fully realized *Yoga* master living on land, Matsyendra, now known as the "king of fishes," shares all that he has learned with his students. Over time these students spread the great teachings of *Yoga* to the whole world.

In addition to these three myths, there are several classical *Yoga* texts that cover the origins, intricacies and benefits of *āsana* in varying degrees of detail. They include the *Haṭha Yoga Pradīpikā*, the *Gheraṇḍa Saṁhitā*, *Yoga Makaranda*, the *Śiva Sūtras*, and the *Yoga Yājñavalkya*.

Our primary references for explaining the practice and purpose of *Yoga āsana* will be Patañjali's *Yoga Sūtras* and the teachings of T. Krishnamacharya, which we feel are the most practical and relevant to modern times. According to the *sūtras*, *āsana* is defined by its qualities, *sthira* (steady) and *sukha* (comfortable), rather than its form. In *āsana, sthira* describes a stable body, steady breathing and a mind that's focused and alert. *Sukha* refers to a comfortable body with smooth breathing and a mind at ease. Linking the breath with movement in our practice helps to ensure that the qualities of *sthira* and *sukha* are maintained.

Patañjali says that with correct practice we develop a stronger body and a sharper mind, capable of clear perception and discernment. Additionally, regular *āsana* practice offers us more resilience and protection from life's ever-changing conditions.

T. Krishnamacharya taught that *āsana* has two major components: structural and energetic. He used the *Pañca Maya* Models and *Prāṇa/Agni/Mala*, among others, for assessing these two components.

To Sum Up:

- References to *āsana* were found in cave drawings over 5000 years ago.
- Though *āsana* is the most popular and recognizable, it is only one of *Yoga's* many tools.
- There are several myths that explain the origins of *āsana*.
- Several classical texts, including the *Haṭha Yoga Pradīpikā* and the *Gheraṇḍa Saṁhitā,* discuss *āsana* in detail.
- Our primary reference for discussing *āsana* are Patañjali's *Yoga Sūtras* and the teachings of T. Krishnamacharya.
- Patañjali defines *āsana* by its qualities, *sthira* and *sukha*, rather than its form.

CHAPTER 9

Yoga's Subtle Anatomy: The *Pañca Maya* Model

If you're having lunch with a close friend, a typical conversation might begin with, "How are you?" Your first response might be, "Life is good!" Then you'd bring each other up to date on health issues, your latest interests and what's going on in your personal and professional relationships. Clearly, the "you" in "How are you?" has many dimensions. Whether or not we're aware of it, we are holistic, multi-faceted human beings.

This same holistic view of the individual was expressed thousands of years ago as the *Vedic Pañca Maya* Model. In Sanskrit, the word "*pañca*" means five, and in this context the word "*maya*" means something that permeates. The *Pañca Maya* Model, which forms the basis of *Yoga*'s subtle anatomy, describes five interconnected aspects of the individual. These *mayas* range from the gross physical level to our most subtle emotional level. Because they are interconnected and permeable, whatever happens at one level always influences the others.

The goal in this model is to achieve and maintain optimum health throughout the system.

Annamaya

The *Annamaya* is our anatomy or physical structure. It includes the skin, bones, tissues, organs and fluids. Based on the teachings of *Yoga* and *Āyurveda*, the three factors for maintaining a healthy body are food, exercise and rest. In *Āyurveda*, food also includes herbs, which are considered superfoods, as well as massage oils, which are viewed as food for the skin.

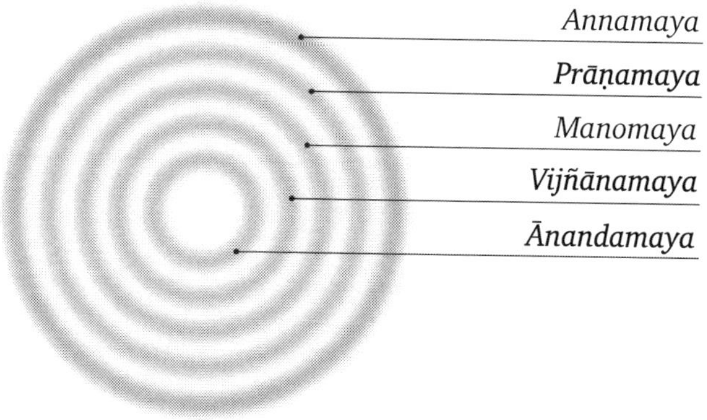

Āyurveda, India's traditional medical system and *Yoga*'s sister science, outlines the following principles of proper nutrition:

- Always eat foods that are fresh, in season, locally grown and, if possible, organic.
- When eating, we should sit down and eat slowly.
- Reduce all distractions.
- Express gratitude for everything and everyone responsible for our meal.

In addition, the science of *Āyurveda* outlines three types of constitutions with specific food and lifestyle guidelines for each.

At the *Annamaya* level, sleep is also essential because of its powerful regenerative effects. *Āyurveda* offers several suggestions to achieve its maximum benefits. We should make an effort to go to bed at approximately the same time every night and get six to eight hours of sleep. Though sleep needs vary based on individual constitution and factors such as illness, stress and stage of life, most adults need to observe these suggestions to function optimally. To this end, we should create proper sleep rituals such as eating our last bite and disconnecting from electronic distractions at least a few hours before bedtime. Eating properly, getting enough exercise and practicing healthy nighttime rituals helps us to reach the state of deep, dreamless sleep the body needs to fully rejuvenate itself.

Yoga's primary tool for a healthy *Annamaya* is the practice of *āsana*. As the spine is the foundation of our anatomy, it is essential to move it regularly in all directions to maintain our strength, flexibility and structural integrity.

Prāṇamaya

The *Prāṇamaya* refers to our physiology. This *maya* consists of all the basic functions necessary for survival, including respiration, elimination, circulation, digestion and communication. Communication is included because, from birth on, the quality of our lives is contingent on the ability to express our needs.

According to *Yoga*, all physiological functions are controlled by *prāṇa*, our vital energy. Breath centered *āsana*, *prāṇāyāma* (conscious breathing) and chanting are *Yoga*'s techniques for enhancing the *Prāṇamaya*. Any practice that promotes slower, deeper breathing activates the subtle energy of the *Prāṇamaya* and strengthens all of our vital functions.

Manomaya

The *Manomaya* refers to our cognitive mind. This *maya* encompasses the entire learning process, including the information we take in through the senses and our ability to remember and utilize what we have learned.

Someone with a healthy *Manomaya* harbors a desire to learn new things and acts on that desire. This might be accomplished by going back to school, learning a new language or taking a cooking class. In *Yoga*, the *Manomaya* tool of chanting sharpens our senses and improves our memory, thus enhancing our ability to learn.

Vijñānamaya

The *Vijñānamaya* is our personality. It refers to our inherent, individual tendencies and personal style. This *maya* also includes our values and beliefs and the ways they are expressed in our life. Someone with a healthy *Vijñānamaya* sets meaningful goals and behaves in a manner consistent with his or her beliefs. *Yoga*'s primary tools for this *maya* are self-reflection, visualization and meditation.

Ānandamaya

The *Ānandamaya* represents our capacity to experience joy. Someone with a healthy *Ānandamaya* has high self-esteem, a positive outlook on life and an underlying sense of optimism and hopefulness. Although it is widely accepted that part of our *Ānandamaya* is preset at birth, *Yoga* teaches that our potential for joy can be enhanced as we grow older. *Yoga*'s strategies for improving our *Ānandamaya* include meditation, seeking out the company of positive people and engaging in activities and relationships that bring us joy.

As previously stated, the *Pañca Maya* is a holistic model, based on the interconnectedness of our body, breath, mind and emotions. For example, extreme or prolonged stress can lead to shallow, irregular breathing which often creates a lack of mental clarity and inability to focus. Any of these conditions could result in confused values and difficulty in making decisions.

Additionally, our emotional state both reflects and affects our posture. We are far more likely to stand straight and tall when we are hopeful and happy and slouch over when we are feeling depressed.

The following story specifically illustrates the cause and effect relationships between the *Maya*s:

Wayne's story:

Wayne is a professional theatre critic who complains of upper back pain and feelings of discontentment. To improve his *Annamaya*, he uses *āsana* to help open the front of his body and relieve his discomfort. While practicing, he notices his breathing is shallow and he lacks energy. As a result of linking his movements with breath and performing *prāṇāyāma*, he experiences increased energy at the *Prāṇamaya* level. Wayne observes that although he now has more vitality, his memory is still poor and he lacks focus at work. To address these *Manomaya* issues, he begins studying French to develop better memory and focus. Still dissatisfied, he realizes he needs to reflect on the source of his discontentment. This *Vijñānamaya* tool of reflection reveals to him that his job is not aligned with his values. While meditating, he visualizes his true dream of being a published poet living in the south of France. He joins a writers group, a community that supports him in doing what he loves, thus deeply fulfilling his *Ānandamaya*.

As this story clearly illustrates, *Yoga* offers tools to work with the whole person, effecting change in all five dimensions of our lives. When we see ourselves through the *Pañca Maya* lens, we are able to choose the appropriate tools to reduce suffering and attain optimum health and more sustained joy at every level.

To Sum Up:

- The *Pañca Maya* Model sees the human system as five interconnected dimensions:
    1. *Annamaya* — physical anatomy
    2. *Prāṇamaya* — physiological functions
    3. *Manomaya* — intellect, cognitive mind, senses
    4. *Vijñānamaya* — personality, inherent tendencies, values
    5. *Ānandamaya* — underlying emotional tone
- *Yoga* and *Āyurveda* offer tools for creating positive change in each of these *mayas*:
    1. *Annamaya* — food, *āsana*, rest
    2. *Prāṇamaya* — breath-centered *āsana*, *prāṇāyāma*, chanting
    3. *Manomaya* — chanting, continued education
    4. *Vijñānamaya* — self-reflection, visualization, meditation
    5. *Ānandamaya* — meditation, cultivating positive interpersonal relationships and engaging in activities that bring us joy

CHAPTER 10

An Energetic Model: *Prāṇa/Agni/Mala*

While *Yoga* offers many tools for self-improvement, the most widely known is the practice of postures (*āsana*). It is in this area we find the greatest variety of techniques, principles and guidelines—all of which can be quite confusing for the beginner. Therefore, before we begin to practice *āsana* or *prāṇāyāma*, we must first understand the holistic, energetic model upon which they are based, the *Prāṇa/Agni/Mala* Model.

The *Prāṇa/Agni/Mala* Model

In ancient times, *Yoga* practices were used primarily to cleanse and purify the human system. The essential tools for purification were (and still are) breath-centered *āsana* and conscious breathing techniques (*prāṇāyāma*). T. Krishnamacharya's *Prāṇa/Agni/Mala* Model is the foundational reference for the correct application of these tools.

Prāṇa is the subtle energy or life-force contained in every living human being. Centered in the chest area, *prāṇa* is affected by the interaction with our external environment, specifically the air we breathe and the food we eat. When *prāṇa* is flowing smoothly throughout the system, the result is abundant health, vitality and optimism.

Agni, located in the center of the torso, is our digestive fire. It is represented as a flame and is responsible for burning our accumulated *mala* (toxins). When the flame of *agni* is burning steadily and brightly, the results are improved digestion, increased resilience, a stronger immune system and a greater passion for living.

Mala, located in the lower abdominal region, is the accumulated waste of a poor diet. In a *Yoga* context, our diet includes not just the food we eat but everything that enters our system through all five senses: sight, hearing, touch, smell and taste—in other words, our entire sensate experience. While foods that are fresh, wholesome and non-processed are the easiest to digest, according to the *Yoga Sūtras*, the most digestible experiences are those with the qualities of honesty, kindness, fairness, moderation and gratitude. Experiences lacking in these qualities remain in the system as toxic residue. Without *yogic* intervention, this toxicity accumulates throughout our life.

How to Activate *Prāṇa/Agni/Mala*

The dynamics of these three functions—*prāṇa*, *agni* and *mala*—are cyclical. A slow, deep inhale activates *prāṇa* much like oxygen fans a flame. This *prāṇa* is drawn downward toward the digestive fire of *agni*, increasing its intensity. This now brightly burning *agni* is then drawn further down toward the *mala,* initiating the purification process.

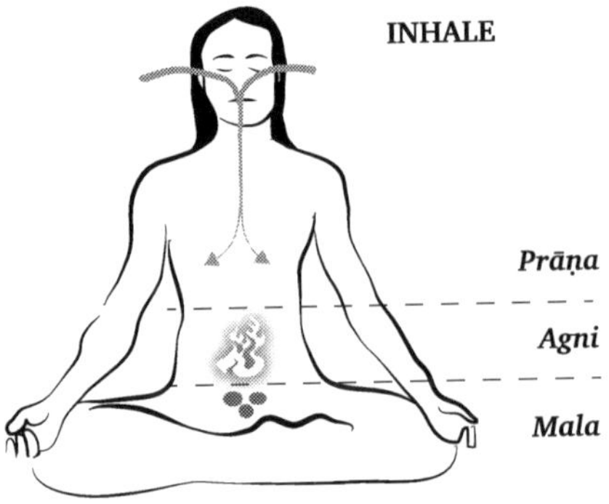

Then, as we take a slow, deep exhale, the abdominal contraction lifts the *mala* toward the *agni,* further burning the accumulated waste. The continued exhale expels the burnt-up residue from the body, completing the purification process.

The *Prāṇa/Agni/Mala* model illustrates the fundamental relationship between breath and movement in the practice of *āsana*. All movements

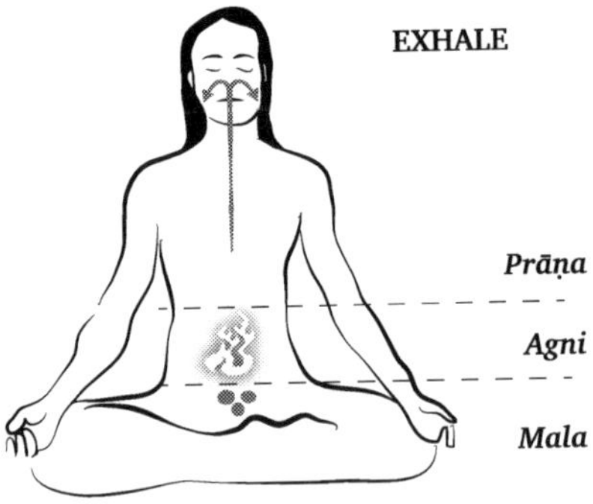

done on exhale move the waste toward the fire; those done on inhale draw the fire toward the waste. Based on this model, it is clear that breath-centered *āsana* and *prāṇāyāma* are powerful tools for purifying the body and mind.

We can choose to look at this model literally or as a metaphor. Either way, understanding the relationship between *prāṇa*, *agni* and *mala* enables us to view our practice from a more energetic perspective and experience increased physical and psychological benefits.

To Sum Up:

- T. Krishnamacharya offered the *Prāṇa/Agni/Mala* Model as the foundation for all *āsana* and *prāṇāyāma* practice.
- This model is energetic, holistic and wellness-based.
- The *Prāṇa/Agni/Mala* Model describes a process of purification based on the proper digestion, assimilation and elimination of our accumulated experience.

CHAPTER 11

The Energetic Effects of Practice: *Bṛṁhana, Laṅghana* and *Samana*

How do you feel at the end of a practice? More energized, more relaxed, perhaps some combination of the two? A competent *Yoga* teacher chooses specific *āsana*, *prāṇāyāma*, visualizations and sounds to create a desired energetic effect. These effects are actually a combination of physical sensations, physiological functions and emotions, created by the flow of energy moving through the body.

Drawing from *Yoga* and *Āyurveda*, T. Krishnamacharya outlined three distinct energetic qualities for guiding a student's practice: *bṛṁhaṇa*, *laṅghana* and *samana*.

The quality of *bṛṁhaṇa* (to energize) heats and tonifies the system. It stimulates alertness in the mind and creates warmth in the body. Poses that open the front of the body, such as backbends and poses linked together in a flowing series (*vinyāsa*), are *bṛṁhaṇa*. In both breath-centered *āsana* and *prāṇāyāma*, inhaling, lengthening the inhale and holding the breath after inhale all promote the *bṛṁhaṇa* effect. Sounds that are loud, high-pitched and fast also create a *bṛṁhaṇa* effect.

By contrast, *laṅghana* (to reduce) cools and relaxes. It decreases agitation in the mind and promotes a feeling of relaxation in the body. Postures that stretch the back, such as forward bends, side stretches and twists, create this effect. Regarding the breath, exhaling, lengthening the exhale and short holds after exhale are all *laṅghana* techniques. Sounds that are soft, low and slow bring about a *laṅghana* effect as well.

Samana (to balance) promotes mental stability and equilibrium in the body. The *samana* effect is created by combining *bṛṁhaṇa* and *laṅghana* postures, such as backbends, forward bends, and twists. It also emphasizes symmetrical postures that straighten the spine. At the level of the breath, *samana* is achieved by equalizing the inhale, exhale and the pauses in between. Sounds that combine *laṅghana* and *bṛṁhaṇa* tones will lead to a *samana* effect.

In order to fully achieve these effects *Yoga's* tools must be appropriately adapted and applied to the individual. This explains why in a group class the same exact practice might be experienced differently and have different effects on each student.

To Sum Up:

- *Yoga* practice manipulates the flow of energy through the body.
- It is possible to feel the effects of this energy both during and after the practice.
- The three energetic effects are:

    1. *bṛṁhaṇa* (heating)
    2. *laṅghana* (relaxing)
    3. *samana* (balancing).

- *Āsana*, *prāṇāyāma*, and sound are the primary tools to create these energetic effects.
- These are general principles; the effects will vary from individual to individual.

"The success of *Yoga* does not lie in the ability to perform postures but in how it positively changes the way we live our life and our relationships."

T.K.V. Desikachar

PART II:
How It Can Work for You

CHAPTER 12

Classification of *Āsana*

The spine is the central focus in *āsana* for several reasons:

- It is the structural core of the body.
- It affects, and is affected by most physical movements.
- It is the nexus for all the nerves carrying messages between the brain and the body.

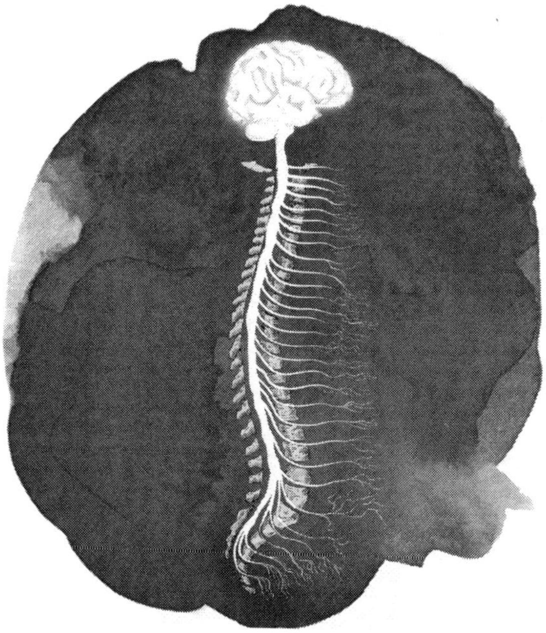

The human spine is capable of moving in five directions: forward, backward, twisting, lateral and inverted. These five directions are the basis for the classifications of all *āsana*. Following are examples of each of these classifications:

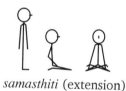

samasthiti (extension)

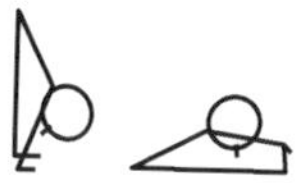

paścimatāna (forward bend)

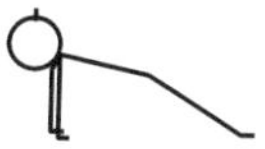

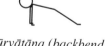

pūrvātāna (backbend)

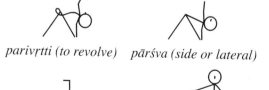

parivṛtti (to revolve)

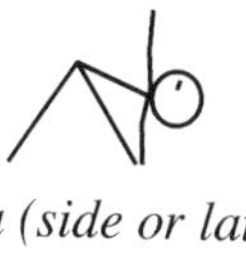

pārśva (side or lateral)

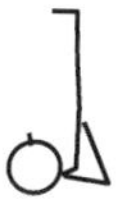

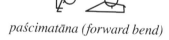

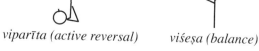

viparīta (active reversal)

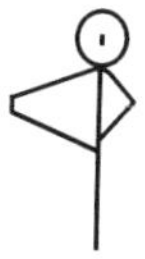

viśeṣa (balance)

Each direction/classification is linked to a variety of physiological functions and specific energetic effects in the body and mind. We will explain each classification and its corresponding postures in terms of three components: form, function and experience.

Form

The first component is form: how the *āsana* looks. Form is a description of the physical profile or shape of the posture. In *Yoga*, there is a relationship between the ideal form of the posture (*prakṛti*) and the actual form a particular individual is capable of achieving on any given day (*vikṛti*).

Although the ideal posture is a standardized form that preserves the image of the pose throughout time, one should only attempt this form if it can be achieved without sacrificing safety, stability and comfort. Otherwise, the posture should be modified to accommodate each individual's unique capabilities and limitations.

Function

The second component is function: what the *āsana* does. It is the anatomical and physiological action of the posture. For example, the function of a twist is the rotation of the spine and the compression of the corresponding organs.

Experience

The last component is experience: how the *āsana* feels. This is highly subjective. Although there is an overall effect to each *āsana* classification, every person will perceive and respond to the posture in his or her own unique way. Experience includes physical sensations as well as energetic, mental and emotional qualities.

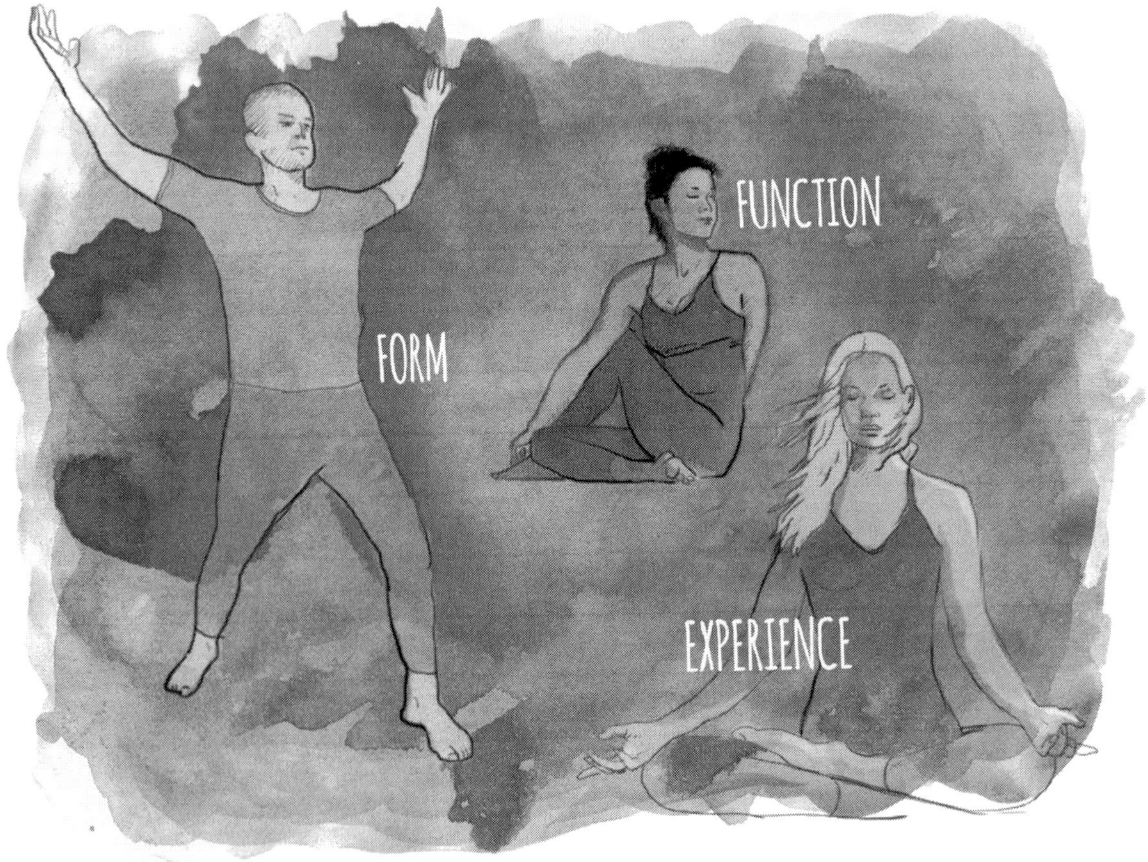

SAMASTHITI, meaning "equal" or "balanced," are symmetrical postures in which the spine is neutral and extended. These are typically done as the first and last poses in a practice.

Here are some *āsanas* in this classification, along with their Sanskrit names.

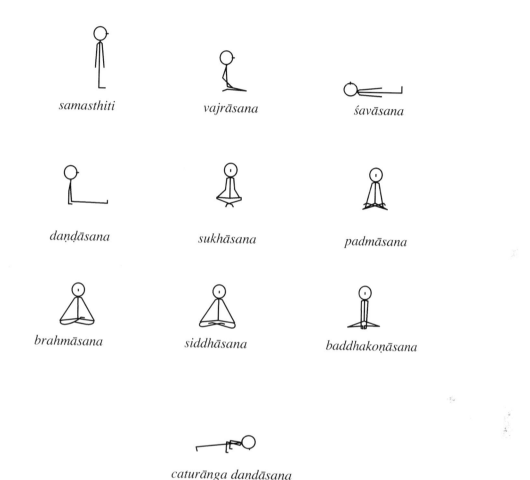

samasthiti

vajrāsana

śavāsana

daṇḍāsana

sukhāsana

padmāsana

brahmāsana

siddhāsana

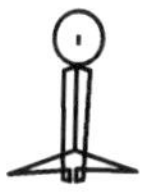

baddhakoṇāsana

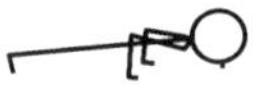

caturānga daṇḍāsana

Following are the form, function and experience of this classification.

Form — Whether sitting, standing or lying down, the spine is straight and fully extended.

Function — These poses increase the space between the vertebrae, creating axial extension and restoring the natural spinal curves. *Samasthiti* postures, which are done on inhale and exhale, build strength and elasticity in the muscles and connective tissues around the spine and rib cage. They also improve postural alignment, thus reducing stress on the whole system and enhancing organ function. Seated *samasthiti* postures are the classical positions for breathing and meditation. Supine *samasthiti* postures, such as *śavāsana*, are used for resting.

Experience — *Samasthiti* postures are used to create a *samana* effect. They promote a feeling of spaciousness and a greater sense of balance and stability.

PAŚCIMATĀNA, meaning "stretching the west" are forward bends. The name refers to the tradition of *Yogis* facing east, toward the rising sun, when practicing. For them, bending forward stretched the back or west side of the body.

Here are some *āsanas* in this classification, along with their Sanskrit names.

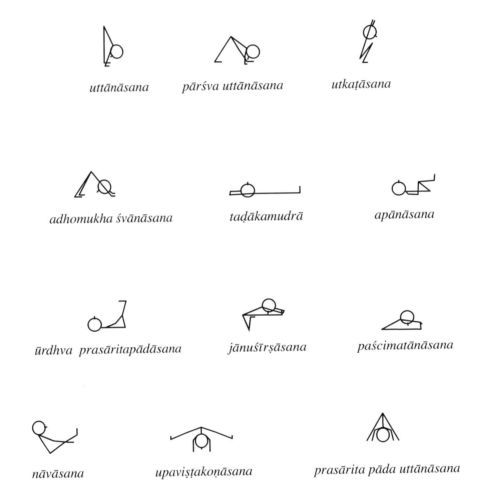

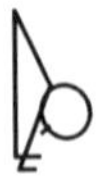
uttānāsana

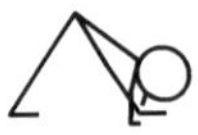
pārśva uttānāsana

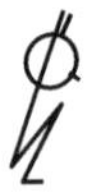
utkaṭāsana

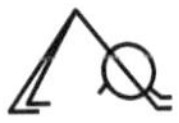
adhomukha śvānāsana

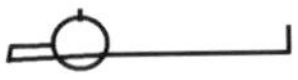
taḍākamudrā

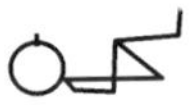
apānāsana

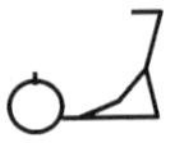
ūrdhva prasāritapādāsana

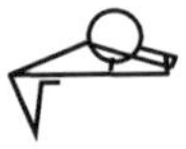
jānuśīrṣāsana

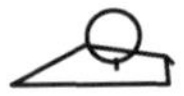
paścimatānāsana

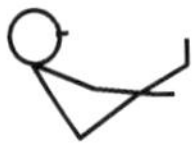
nāvāsana

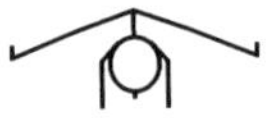
upaviṣṭakoṇāsana

prasārita pāda uttānāsana

Following are the form, function and experience of this classification.

Form — Whether standing, sitting, supine or kneeling, *paścimatāna* is the movement of either the torso toward the legs or the legs toward the torso.

Function — *Paścimatāna* stretches and strengthens the lumbosacral spine, the erector spinae muscles and the upper back and neck. Always done on exhale or pause after exhale, *paścimatāna* increases the contraction in the abdominal region, lengthening both the exhale and the inhale. In general, these postures are designed to increase strength and flexibility, reduce structural asymmetry and improve the overall alignment of the body.

Experience — *Paścimatāna* postures are used to create a *laṅghana* effect. Done on exhale, forward bends promote a sense of calmness, release and a quieter mind. In addition, there is a feeling of lengthening in the back of the body.

***PŪRVĀTĀNA**, meaning* "stretching the east" are backbends. Traditionally, because the practitioner was facing the sun they created a feeling of warmth and openness in the body.

Here are some *āsanas* in this classification, along with their Sanskrit names.

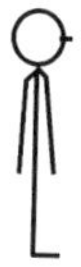

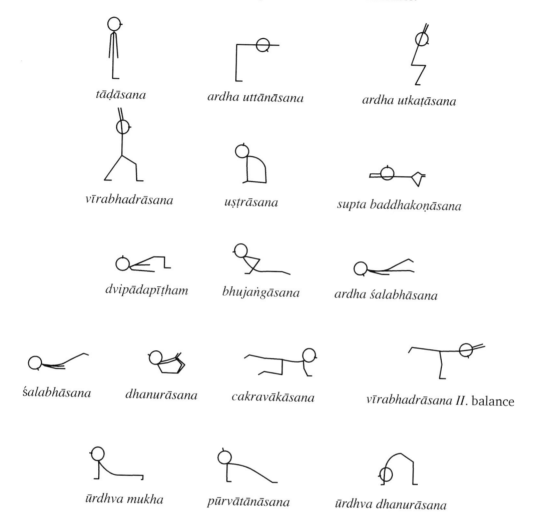

tāḍāsana

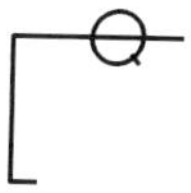

ardha uttānāsana

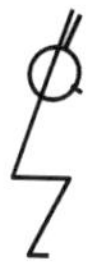

ardha utkaṭāsana

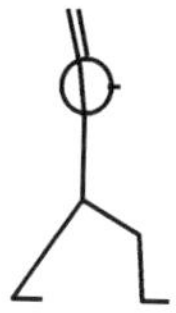

vīrabhadrāsana

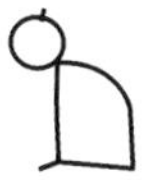

uṣṭrāsana

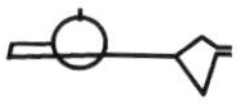

supta baddhakoṇāsana

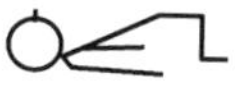

dvipādapīṭham

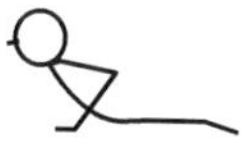

bhujaṅgāsana

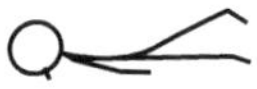

ardha śalabhāsana

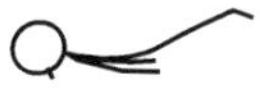

śalabhāsana

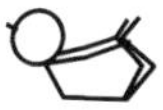

dhanurāsana

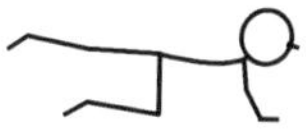

cakravākāsana

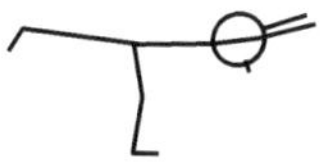

vīrabhadrāsana II. balance

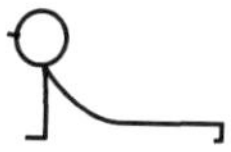

ūrdhva mukha

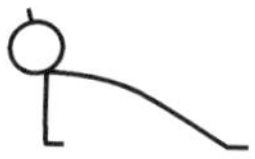

pūrvātānāsana

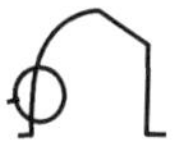

ūrdhva dhanurāsana

Following are the form, function and experience of this classification.

Form — In *pūrvātāna* poses, whether standing, prone (lying on the belly), kneeling or supine, the back is arched and the torso is moving away from the legs.

Function — *Pūrvātāna* postures expand the chest, stretch the intercostal muscles, solar plexus, abdomen, psoas, hips and thighs while contracting the back. They also create space for the diaphragm to move freely. Backbends decompress the organs in the front of the body and gently compress the kidneys. They can reduce thoracic kyphosis (rounded upper back) while strengthening the back muscles and shoulder girdle. Done on inhale the chest expands allowing for a deeper, more diaphragmatic breath.

Experience — *Pūrvātāna* postures are used to create a *bṛṁhaṇa* effect. Done on inhale, backbends promote a feeling of increased heat and energy. In addition, *pūrvātāna* poses are felt as an openness in the front of the body.

PARIVṚTTI, meaning "to revolve," are twisting postures. Much like wringing the water out of a cloth, these postures squeeze the internal organs, facilitating the reduction of toxins or *mala*.

Here are some *āsanas* in this classification, along with their Sanskrit names.

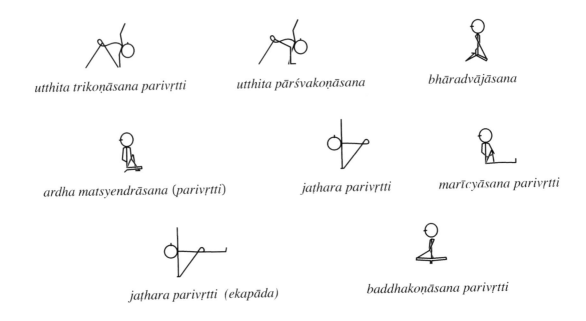

utthita trikoṇāsana parivṛtti

utthita pārśvakoṇāsana

bhāradvājāsana

ardha matsyendrāsana (parivṛtti)

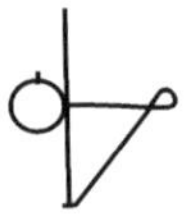

jaṭhara parivṛtti

marīcyāsana parivṛtti

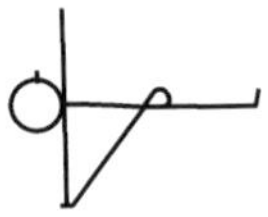

jaṭhara parivṛtti (ekapāda)

baddhakoṇāsana parivṛtti

Following are the form, function and experience of this classification.

Form — Whether standing, sitting or supine, *parivṛtti* poses twist the spine around a fixed point of the body.

Function — *Parivṛtti* poses create rotation of the spinal vertebrae, working both the deep and superficial muscles of the spine and abdomen. Done on exhale, twists emphasize the relationship between the pelvis, shoulders and spine. They reduce structural asymmetry, help maintain intervertebral elasticity and stimulate respiratory, digestive and eliminative functions. *Parivṛtti*, like all asymmetrical postures, help with right-left brain integration and physical balance.

Experience — *Parivṛtti* postures are used to create a *laṅghana* effect. Done on exhale, twists create a feeling of turning, squeezing and stretching in the torso. The result is a sense of release and relaxation.

PĀRŚVA, meaning "side" or "lateral," are asymmetrical postures that stretch the sides of the body. They have a lengthening effect on one side and a feeling of compression on the other.

Here are some *āsanas* in this classification, along with their Sanskrit names.

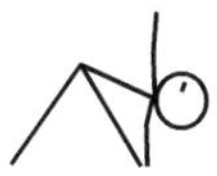

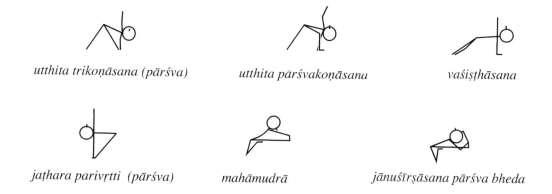

utthita trikoṇāsana (pārśva)

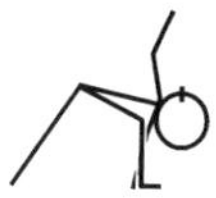

utthita pārśvakoṇāsana

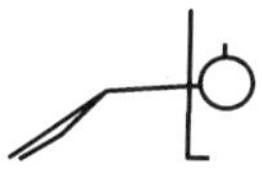

vaśiṣṭhāsana

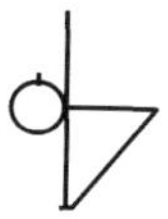

jaṭhara parivṛtti (pārśva)

mahāmudrā

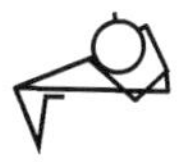

jānuśīrṣāsana pārśva bheda

Following are the form, function and experience of this classification.

Form — Whether standing, sitting or supine, *pārśva* postures move the spine laterally.

Function — *Pārśva* poses flex the spine, stretching the torso from shoulder to hip. In laterals, we alternately stretch and contract the intercostal, erector and quadratus muscles on each side of the body. These poses reduce structural asymmetry and maintain intervertebral elasticity. As with any asymmetrical postures, lateral poses help integrate both sides of the brain.

Experience — Once again *pārśva* postures can be performed on either inhale or exhale. On inhale, they create a *bṛṁhaṇa* effect and on exhale, *laṅghana*. Laterals also produce a feeling of openness on the extended side of the torso.

VIPARĪTA are inversions. With the legs higher than the heart and the heart higher than the head, inversions use the reverse pull of gravity to cleanse the lower half of the body and more easily oxygenate the upper half.

Here are some *āsanas* in this classification, along with their Sanskrit names.

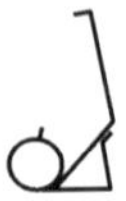

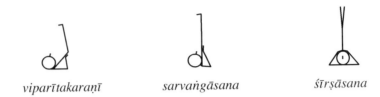

viparītakaraṇī

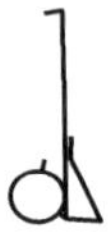

sarvaṅgāsana

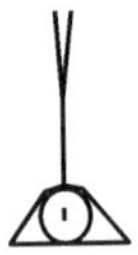

śīrṣāsana

(The above poses are progressive. If you can't do the first, you can't do the second; if you can't do the second, you shouldn't try the third.)

Following are the form, function and experience of this classification.

Form — In *viparīta* poses, the legs are higher than the heart and the heart is higher than the head.

Function — The spine is vertical in these postures, reversing the pull of gravity. Done on either inhale or exhale, inversions integrate the spinal curves and improve respiration. *Viparīta* postures extend and strengthen the upper body, abdomen, neck and torso. Inversions are the only poses where the hips have freedom of movement.

Experience — The effect of inversions can either be *bṛṁhaṇa* or *laṅghana*. Although initially disorienting, they ultimately create a feeling of stability and spaciousness.

Inversions are extreme postures with numerous benefits. Because of the many potential dangers you should always have the guidance of a competent teacher when attempting *viparīta* poses. There are many conditions that make inversions difficult and potentially harmful. Therefore they **should be avoided if** any of the following conditions are present:

- epilepsy
- cervical disc problem
- high blood pressure
- glaucoma
- during menstruation
- during pregnancy

VIŚEṢA, meaning special, is a category of postures that includes arm and leg balances. Depending on the *āsana*, *viśeṣa* poses are done on inhale, exhale or hold after exhale. This classification is far more physically demanding than all the others and has, traditionally, been used to build confidence in younger students. Because children are far more resilient than adults, *viśeṣa* places less emphasis than other poses on breathing, adaptation, individualization and concern for injury. In this category, greater emphasis is placed on perfection of the form, which, combined with increased difficulty, provides a strong focus for the developing mind of a child. This category does not conform to the *Prāṇa/Agni/Mala* Model.

Here are some *āsanas* in this classification, along with their Sanskrit names.

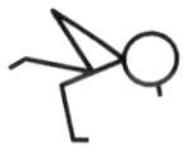

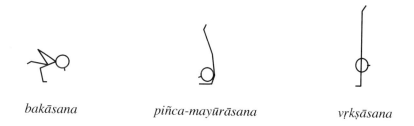

bakāsana

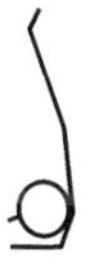

piñca-mayūrāsana

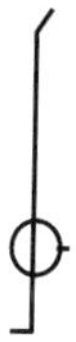

vṛkṣāsana

Positive Aspects of *Viśeṣa* Postures

They:

- help increase focus.
- build confidence in both children and adults.
- help us better handle the challenges of life.
- are lighthearted and fun, adding variety to our practice.
- offer intense physical challenge.
- improve strength, balance and stamina.
- demonstrate the range and potential of the human body.

Negative Aspects of *Viśeṣa* Postures

They:

- cause shallow, irregular breathing.
- carry high potential for injury.
- can be mentally destabilizing.
- erode confidence if unable to perform *āsana*.
- promote unhealthy comparison and competitiveness.
- confuse people as to the purpose of *āsana*.

MULTI-FUNCTION POSTURES. While most postures function within their own classification, there are some *āsana* that fit in more than one category. Because these poses fulfill more than one function, they are highly beneficial. For instance, *pārśva uttānāsana* combines a forward bend (*paścimatāna*) with a slight twist (*parivṛtti*) and a side stretch (*pārśva*).

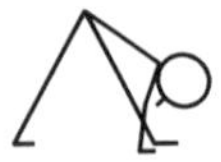

pārśva uttānāsana

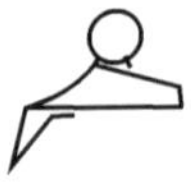

mahāmudrā

In *mahāmudrā* we bend forward, with both hands on the foot (*paścimatāna*) and the back slightly arched (*pūrvātāna*); then, we simultaneously extend the spine (*samasthiti*) and drop the chin.

To Sum Up:

- There are seven classifications of *āsana*:

  1. ***Samasthiti*** (equal) are always symmetrical and begin and end the practice. They extend the spine and are done on both inhale and exhale. They create the feeling of being taller and lighter.

  2. ***Paścimatāna*** (forward bends) can be either symmetrical or asymmetrical. They stretch the back of the body and are always done on exhale. The resulting feeling is one of relaxation.

  3. ***Pūrvātāna*** (backbends) can also be both symmetrical and asymmetrical. They stretch the front of the body and are primarily done on inhale. They create a feeling of increased alertness and energy.

  4. ***Parivṛtti*** (twists) are always asymmetrical. They rotate the spine and are done on exhale. Coming out of these postures creates a feeling of release.

  5. ***Pārśva*** (side) are always asymmetrical, as well. They are lateral poses that stretch the side of the body and are done on exhale. They create a feeling of more space and length in the torso.

  6. ***Viparīta*** (inversion) can be symmetrical or asymmetrical. They stretch and strengthen the body, open the hips and can be done on inhale or exhale. Depending on the pose, they can create a feeling of relaxation or increased energy.

  7. ***Viśeṣa*** (balance) can also be either symmetrical or asymmetrical. They increase strength and balance and can be done on inhale, exhale or hold after exhale. They create a feeling of confidence, energy and a sense of accomplishment.

- Some poses are combinations of different classifications and fulfill more than one function.

CHAPTER 13

Breath and Movement: Fundamentals of *Āsana*

Most modern practitioners equate *Yoga* with *āsana* (postures), often using the words interchangeably. In reality, *Yoga* is both a philosophy and a complete holistic system of healing which addresses the needs of the body, breath and mind. *Āsana* is only one of its many tools. In our experience, when we explore the relationship between attention and breath and movement, *āsana* becomes a truly integrative experience.

The breath serves as powerful barometer for our mental, emotional and physical states. Patañjali adds that when our *āsana* is breath-centered, we are far more likely to apply the appropriate effort needed to create and maintain a relaxed body and a quiet steady mind. *Āsana* is elevated from a purely physical exercise to a far more meditative experience.

According to T. Krishnamacharya, *āsana* is *nava śarīra saṁskāra*, "new body patterns." Initially, the practice of *āsana* creates an awareness of the neuromuscular tendencies that no longer serve us, such as a jutting chin, slouching shoulders or a rounded upper back. In time, appropriate practice creates healthy new patterns, such as keeping the spine tall and the head straight and level.

In this chapter, we will discuss how to approach *āsana* as one part of a complete, holistic healing system, rather than as an isolated physical practice.

Relationship between Breath and Movement

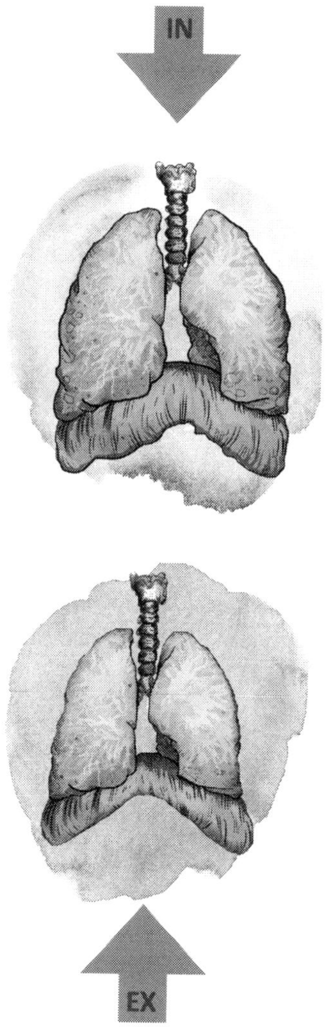

The Dynamics of Breathing

First let's look at the dynamics of breathing. As we inhale, the lungs fill with air and the diaphragm, the principle muscle of breathing, moves downward. On exhale, the diaphragm moves back up into place. Simply put, the inhale is a downward movement from chest to belly. The exhale is an upward movement from belly to chest. In *Yoga āsana*, we will learn to breathe into the lower third of the lungs to create more strength and elasticity in the diaphragm, making each breath deeper and stronger. Diaphragmatic breathing oxygenates the blood more efficiently, improving brain and organ function, as well as activating the relaxation response, thus reducing stress.

In daily life, we are unaware of how we breathe, how we move, and the link between the two. Conscious diaphragmatic breathing lengthens the breath and extends the spine, which assists in the performance of *āsana* and increases its benefits. When we inhale and direct our attention to lifting and expanding the chest, the spine naturally extends. When we exhale and focus on drawing the navel toward the spine, the lower back is supported and lengthened. In addition, consciously directing attention increases awareness of both the movements and the effects of the postures.

Once the relationship between inhale and exhale is established, we begin to practice another component of the complete breath, the pauses. Just as there is a moment of stillness between the swings of a pendulum, there is a natural pause, one or two seconds, between the inhale and exhale.

Synchronizing Breath and Movement

The next step in learning how to integrate breath and movement is a technique called *ujjāyī* (throat breathing). To do *ujjāyī*, breathe through the nose with the mouth closed, constrict the glottis (vocal cords) and make a whispering sound with the breath. This sound is similar to the one we make as we are falling asleep. To experience this breathing technique, lie on your back with your chin slightly tucked and your mouth closed. For many people this position involuntarily constricts the glottis, creating *ujjāyī* breath. This technique, when properly performed, simultaneously lengthens the breath, provides us with a point of focus and helps promote the qualities of *sthira* (steady) and *sukha* (comfortable).

Here are simple steps for learning to synchronize the breath with movement while sitting in a chair, as a preparation for doing so in *āsana*.

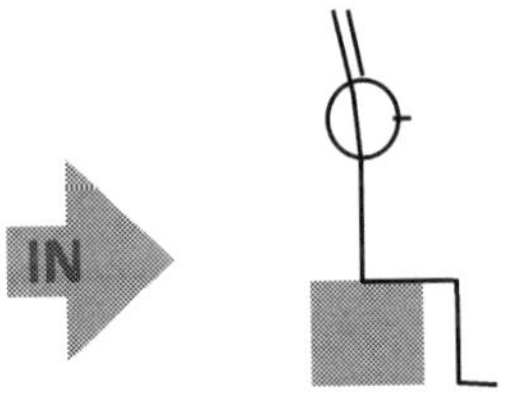

- Take a few *ujjāyī* breaths before beginning.
- Inhale *ujjāyī* while raising your arms up over your head.
- At the end of the inhale, pause the breath and stop the movement for one or two seconds.
- Exhale *ujjāyī* while lowering your arms back to your sides.
- At the end of the exhale, pause the breath and stop the movement for one or two seconds.
- Repeat the movement four to six times.
- Note: Remember to match the speed of your breath with the speed of the movement.

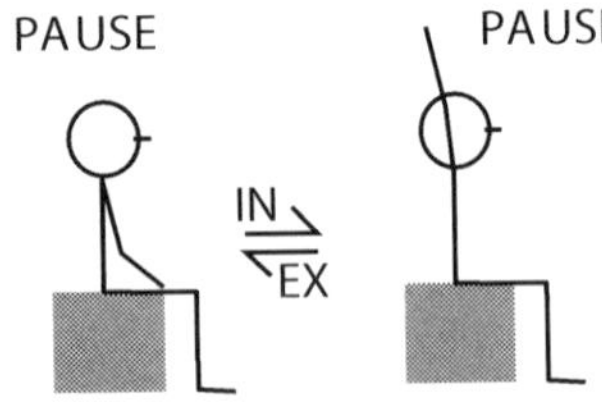

Repetition and Stay

The next components in breath centered *āsana* are repetition and stay, using postures dynamically and statically. In this process, we repeat the *āsana*, synchronizing the *ujjāyī* breath with movement, several times before staying in the pose.

- There are many essential reasons to perform *āsana* in this way. Dynamic movement:
- gives us the opportunity to observe our starting point and how change occurs through repetition.
- warms up the body.
- reduces the possibility for injury.
- increases our range of movement.
- reinforces the synchronization of breath and movement.
- provides feedback on our physical comfort, the quality of our breathing and our focus.
- prepares the body to stay in the posture.
- intensifies the experience and effects of the *āsana*.

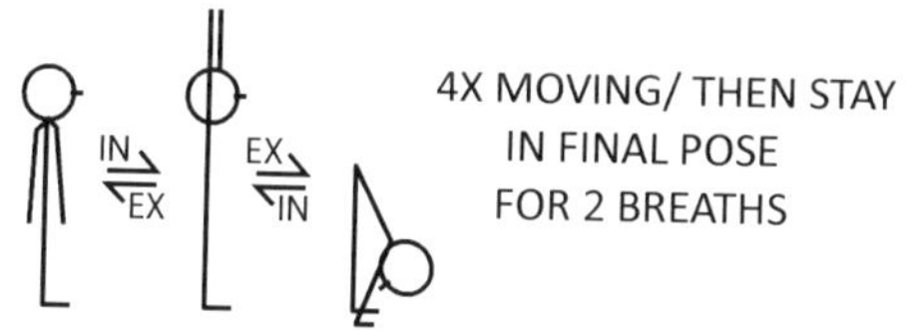

uttānāsana

After enough repetitions to warm up the body without fatiguing it (generally three to six times), the body is now prepared to stay in the pose. The length of time you stay should range from three to six *ujjāyī* breaths. The breath is a reliable gauge for appropriate effort, our physical comfort and state of mind. If your breathing becomes short, shallow or irregular, it's a sign to come out of the pose. You can force the body, you can trick the mind, but the breath never lies.

Now that we have discussed *āsana*'s fundamental principles, the following practice will help you to experience them for yourself.

PRACTICE:

1. Lie on your back, place your hands just above your belly button and notice your natural breath.

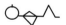

Begin *ujjāyī* breathing while observing the rise and fall of your chest and abdomen. Maintain *ujjāyī* throughout the entire practice. Take 4 breaths. (If *ujjāyī* is not possible breathe in a manner comfortable for you.)

2. Place the arms by your side palms down.

Inhale while raising both arms overhead to the floor behind you. Pause.

Exhale while lowering the arms back down to your sides. Pause.

Repeat 6x (6 times). Rest.

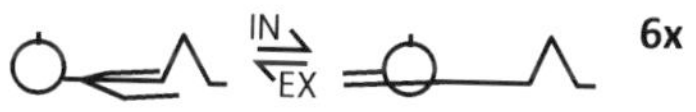

3. Slowly come to your hands and knees.

Place your hands under your shoulders and your knees under your hips, hip width apart.

As you inhale, lift your chest while keeping your chin in a neutral position. Pause.

As you exhale, draw your navel in, while simultaneously moving your hips back towards your heels, bending the elbows and lowering your head. Pause.

Inhale back to starting position. Repeat 6x

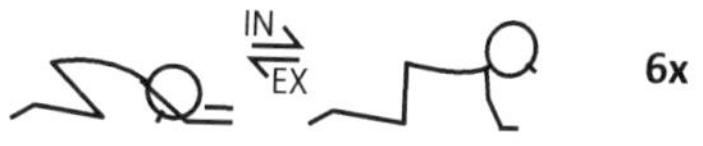

cakravākāsana

4. Slowly come to standing.

- Stand, feet hip width apart. Take a few *ujjāyī* breaths.

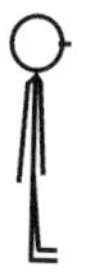

samasthiti

5. On inhale, raise your arms above your head. Pause.

As you exhale, draw the navel in as you lower your arms. Pause. Repeat 6x.

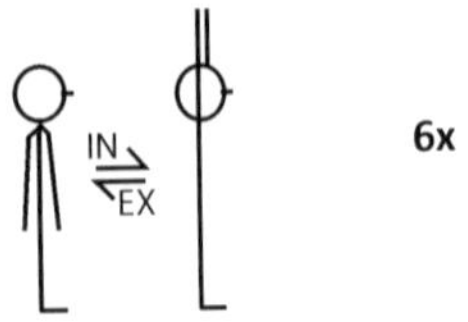

samasthiti

6. Rest.

samasthiti

Take a moment to notice how this simple practice of synchronizing breath and movement has warmed up the body, lengthened the breath and steadied the mind.

To Sum Up:

- *Āsana* is defined by the qualities of *sthira* (stability) and *sukha* (comfort).
- *Āsana* creates awareness of neuromuscular patterns and helps to create new ones.
- Diaphragmatic breathing lengthens the breath, oxygenates the blood and increases the relaxation response.
- *Ujjāyī* breathing lengthens the breath, provides us with a point of focus and helps promote the qualities of *sthira* and *sukha* in *āsana*.
- Synchronizing breath with movement elevates *āsana* from a physical practice to a meditative experience.
- Repetition and stay is a foundational principle of *āsana* practice.

CHAPTER 14

Sequencing Part I: Components of Sequencing

To bake a cake, we begin with a recipe that includes a list of ingredients. When we combine these ingredients in the proper order, the result is the perfect dessert. In designing a *Yoga* practice, the same principle applies. Following are the various components of sequencing required to make the delicious cake of practice:

- intention
- considerations
- classification of *āsana*
- orientations
- reference poses
- transitions
- counterposes
- rests

Intention

Before we begin to design the sequence of any *āsana* practice, it is essential to know our goal or intention. There are many reasons we might choose to do a practice, including one or more of the following:

- to be able to perform a specific *āsana*
- to realize a posture's benefits, including: more strength, greater flexibility, better breathing, relief from pain, improved balance or higher self-esteem
- to create a desired energetic effect, such as: increased vitality, deeper relaxation or feelings of serenity
- to be able to do something tomorrow that we can't do today.

Considerations

For the second component, considerations, we should take into account our immediate needs as well as our long-term goals. In addition, T. Krishnamacharya offered a more extensive list of practical considerations when sequencing our practice. They are:

- *kāla* — time (time of day, season or length of practice)
- *deśa* — location (climate, altitude and general ambience)
- *vayah* — age, stage of life
- *vṛtti* — activities (job, hobbies, responsibilities)
- *śakti* — overall stamina, current energy level, *Āyurvedic* constitution
- *icchā* — depth of commitment, intensity of desire

Here's an example of the considerations of practice. Two different individuals want a personal practice to help reduce their back pain. The first is a vibrant, 16-year-old student who lives on the beach and loves to surf. The other is an overworked, 60-year-old carpenter living in the city. The student is eager to do his practice first thing in the morning, while the carpenter reluctantly agrees to do a short practice before bedtime.

Both individuals have the same desire (*icchā*) to reduce their back pain. However, based on the diversity of their ages (*vayah*), professions and activities (*vṛtti*), they have dramatically different energy levels (*śakti*). These factors, combined with where they live (*deśa*), and their available time (*kāla*), will lead to a very different practice for each.

Classification of *Āsana*

Once we are clear about our intention and considerations, we need to look at the third component, classification of *āsana*. These classifications are based on the direction of movement of the spine. Because each direction of movement has a different form, function and experience, we must only choose postures in the classifications which are essential for achieving our goal. For example, if our goal is a seated twist, there is no need for inversions or laterals.

Once again, the seven classifications are:

- *samasthiti* (extension)
- *paścimatāna* (forward bend)
- *pūrvātāna* (backbend)
- *parivṛtti* (to revolve/twist)
- *pārśva* (side or lateral)
- *viparīta* (inversion)
- *viśeṣa* (balance)

Orientations

There are six possible orientations (the position of the body in space relative to the ground), in

Classification	Orientation					
	Standing	Supine	Prone	Seated	Inverted	Kneeling
Samasthiti (Extension)	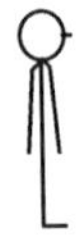	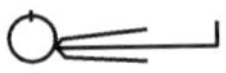		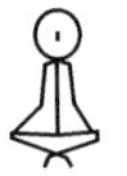		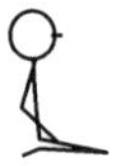
Paścimatāna (Forward Bend)	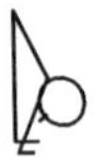	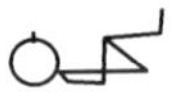		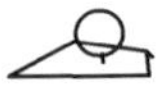	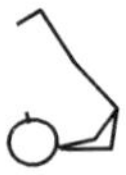	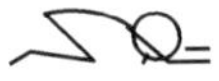
Pūrvātāna (Backbend)	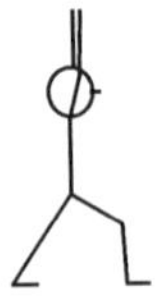	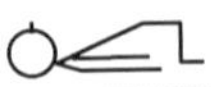	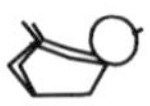	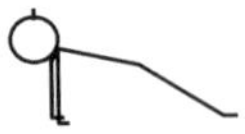		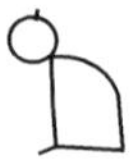
Pārśva (Lateral)	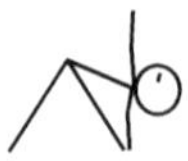	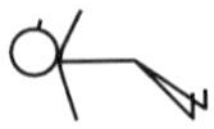		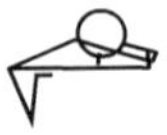		
Parivṛtti (Twist)	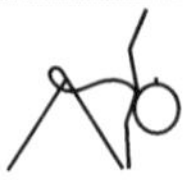			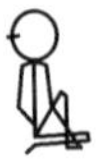		
Viparīta (Inversion)					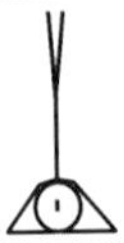	

which *āsana* is performed. The table on page 70 shows most of the classifications of *āsana* that can be done in more than one orientation. T. Krishnamacharya taught the following order of orientation to perform *āsana*:

Standing – Supine – Inverted – Prone – Seated – Kneeling

Here is the logic behind this order:

Standing — Standing postures are the most common position for healthy human beings. They offer the greatest freedom of movement in all directions: extension, forward bend, backbend, lateral bend and twist. Starting a practice from a standing position prepares the entire body for all subsequent postures.

Supine — After vigorous standing postures, lying on the back provides a period of rest and recovery for the body and breath. It also places us in the proper orientation to prepare for inverted postures.

Inverted — Because inverted postures place the body upside down, they create a novel sensation and a new body pattern. Inversions also possess the greatest potential for directing the *agni* (digestive fire) toward the *mala* (residue).

Prone — Lying on the stomach allows us to perform deep backbends and offers the compensation needed after performing inversions.

Kneeling — Kneeling postures are often used as a transition from standing to supine or from prone to seated. They usually serve as compensation for back arches performed on the belly.

Seated — Seated postures are performed after supine or kneeling postures. This orientation requires strength in the back and flexibility in the legs and hips. They are placed at the end of the practice and, if necessary, performed sitting on a chair or using a wall to support the back. When we are able to sit comfortably, seated postures are best used for *prāṇāyāma* and meditation practices.

These orientations provide a foundation for understanding T. Krishnamacharya's sequencing model. It is also possible to start a practice kneeling or lying on the back depending on the student's or group's needs. Following, are some of the many possibilities for different sequencing orientations:

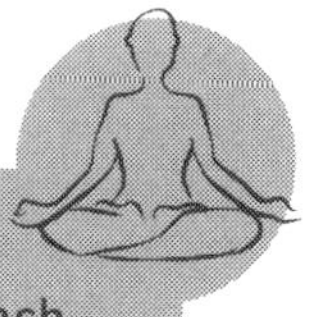

- Knees – Standing – Knees – Stomach – Back – Sitting
- Knees – Stomach – Knees – Stand – Knees – Back – Inversion – Stomach – Back or Knees – Sitting
- Standing – Knees –Back – Stomach – Back – Sitting
- Back – Stomach – Knees – Standing – Knees – Back– Sitting
- Back – Stomach – Knees – Back

Although there are numerous other possibilities for sequencing orientations, T. Krishnamacharya's principles, which are based on an intuitive logic and deep respect for the individual, should be followed whenever possible.

Reference Poses

All reference postures are symmetrical positions in the *samasthiti* classification. We use these simple poses to verify a person's ability to perform *āsana* in a specific orientation. They arc: standing, lying on the back (supine), lying on the stomach (prone), seated and kneeling.

If one is unable to perform the reference posture, they should not attempt any poses in that orientation. For example, if you are unable to stand, you would not perform any standing postures, and if you are unable to lie on your stomach, prone postures are not possible.

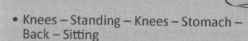

Following are the reference postures for each physical orientation.

Our ability to perform reference postures provides us with a clear guideline for appropriate practice. In addition, they are always the first and last positions in each orientation of the practice. For example, before transitioning from standing to kneeling in a practice, you should return to the standing reference pose.

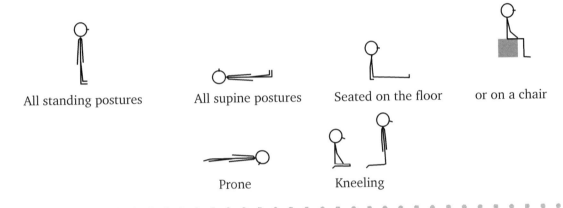

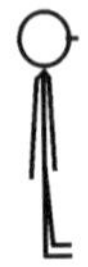

All standing postures

All supine postures

Seated on the floor

or on a chair

Prone

Kneeling

Transitions

Although there are only eight musical notes in a major scale, how we choose to arrange them determines the melody, tempo and, ultimately, the feeling we get from a piece of music. In a *Yoga* practice, the transition from one direction of movement to the next determines its safety, effectiveness and experience. Practices designed with correct transitions achieve the desired result with efficiency, elegance and ease.

Transitions determine the structure and flow of the practice, and it is essential to perform them in the appropriate order. Students are often eager to try all the postures in all their various directions and orientations. While this enthusiasm is essential for sustained practice, problems occur when practitioners choose postures randomly or without knowing the principles for proper sequencing.

The following "Wheel of Transition" model illustrates the correct, time-tested principles for insuring maximum comfort, elegance, efficiency and safety in your practice.

Simply put, before we change the direction of movement (backbend, lateral, twist) in any orientation (standing, seated, etc.), we must create a smooth transition by performing a symmetrical forward bend (SFB) in that same orientation.

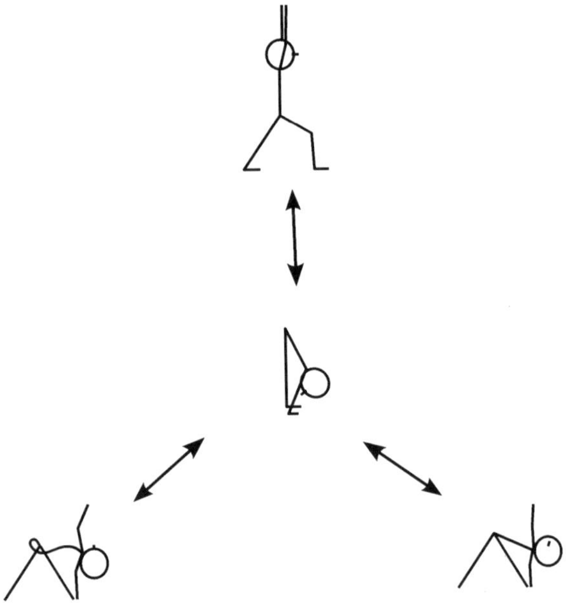

This "Wheel of Transition" illustrates the correct use of a forward bend in the center and the other directions of movement around it.

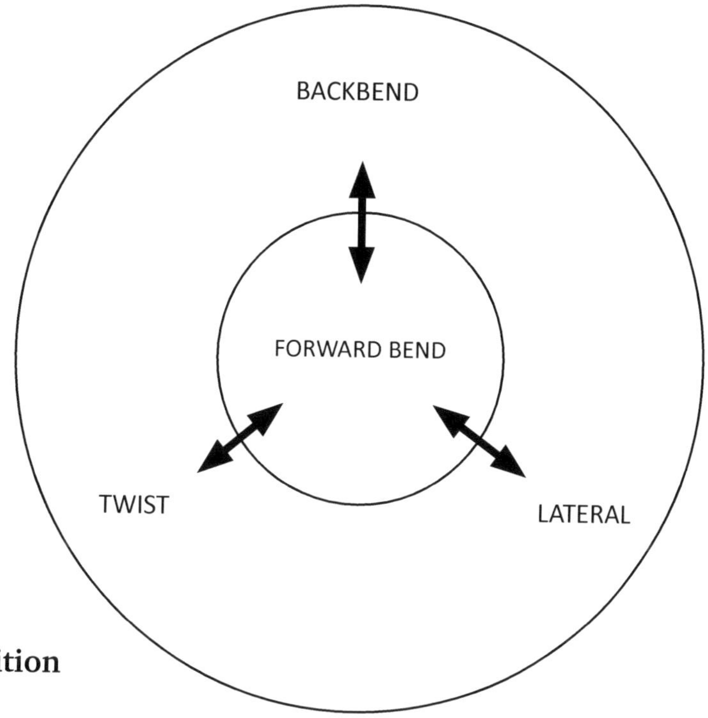

Wheel of Transition

For example:

- Do a symmetrical forward bend (SFB) when going from a backbend to a twist or from a twist to a backbend.

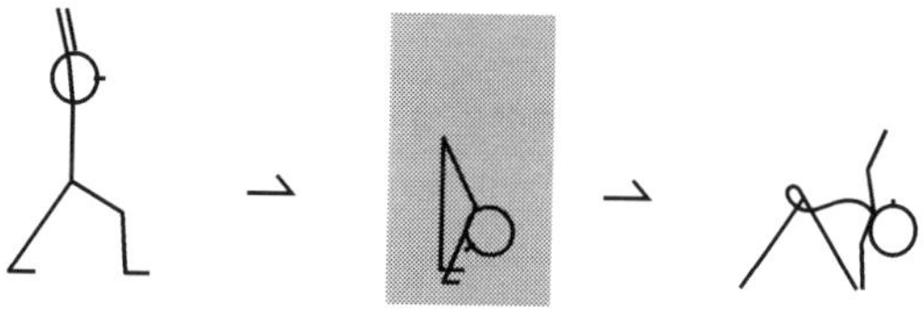

- Do a SFB when going from a twist to a lateral or from a lateral to a twist.

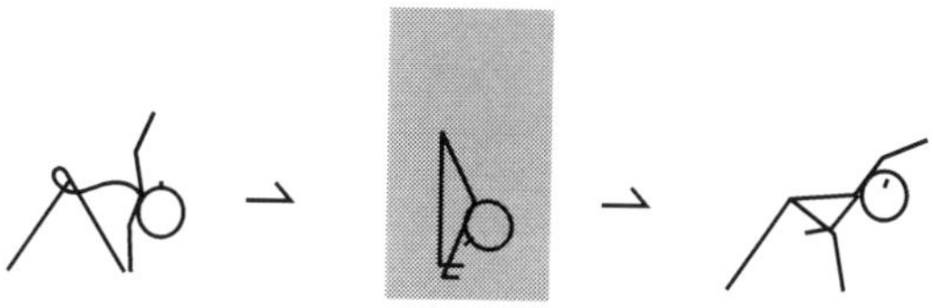

- Do a SFB when going from a backbend to a lateral or from a lateral to a twist.

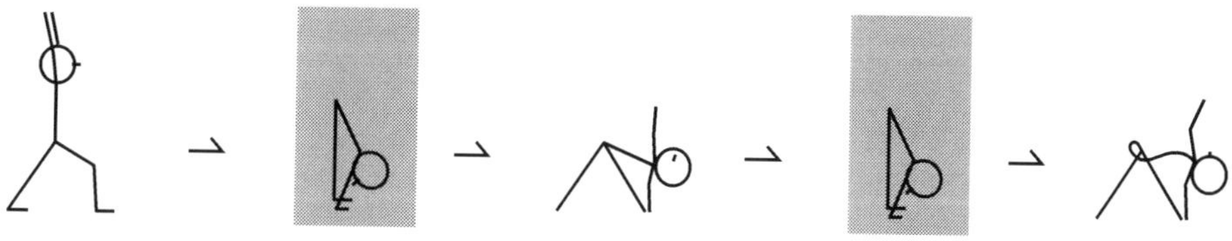

Applying this model brings the body back to a neutral state between each orientation. Ultimately correct transitioning creates a sense of balance, fluidity and enjoyment.

Counterposes

Counterposes (*pratikriyāsana*) are needed to minimize the negative effects of *Yoga āsana* and maximize the positive benefits. These are postures, placed strategically throughout the practice, which bring the body back to neutral, thus preparing us for the next posture.

In general, counterposes are:

- done in the same orientation as the previous pose.
- performed immediately after the pose they are counterposing.
- symmetrical.
- performed dynamically.
- easier than the pose for which they are compensating.

Counterposes have many benefits, including:

- reducing any stress placed on the body from the previous postures.
- minimizing the possibility of injury.
- creating smooth, elegant transitions throughout the practice.
- preparing the body for the following posture.
- returning the body, breath and mind to a state of stability, balance and neutrality.
- enhancing the overall effect and experience of the practice.

Rests

Rests, the suspension of movement, are always taken in a neutral position. For example, *samasthiti* is a rest for standing postures, while lying on the back is a rest for supine or seated. Although *śavāsana* is often the final resting pose, shorter rests are always appropriate throughout the practice, particularly when changing orientations.

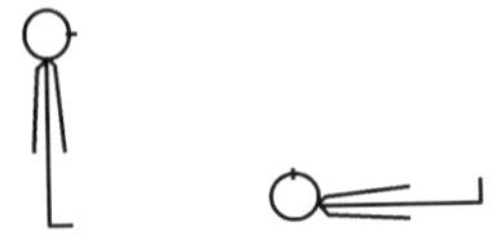

samasthiti *śavāsana*

Rests serve several important functions. They can:

- release or minimize any residual physical strain.
- allow the breath to return to normal.
- help to integrate the effects of the posture.
- increase our ability to observe and reflect.

The eight components of sequencing outlined in this chapter are the building blocks which give *āsana* greater depth and dimensionality. In the next chapter, we will learn how to use these components to create individualized sequences that are comprehensive, elegant and effective.

To Sum Up:

- There are eight components for sequencing a practice:
  1. intention
  2. considerations
  3. classification of *āsana*
  4. orientations
  5. reference poses
  6. transitions
  7. counterposes
  8. rests

- T. Krishnamacharya offered a list of six practical considerations when sequencing our practice:
  1. *kāla* — time (time of day, season or length of practice)
  2. *deśa* — location (climate, altitude and general ambience)
  3. *vayah* — age, stage of life
  4. *vṛtti* — activities (job, hobbies, responsibilities)
  5. *śakti* — stamina, energy level, constitution
  6. *icchā* — degree of commitment, intensity of desire
- T. Krishnamacharya taught the following classical order of orientation to perform *āsana*:
  1. standing
  2. supine
  3. inverted
  4. prone
  5. kneeling
  6. seated

CHAPTER 15

Sequencing, Part II: Designing an *Āsana* Practice

Vinyāsa krama (taking small, logical steps toward a chosen destination) is a core principle in *Yoga* which can be applied to achieving any goal in life. In *āsana* practice, this term has three specific definitions:

- the steps taken to perform each *āsana*, as previously discussed in the chapter on breath and movement (see chapter13).
- the correct arrangement of postures to achieve a goal within a single practice.
- the careful planning of progressive practices to achieve a specific goal over time.

The Stages of Practice

Every season, meal and well-told story has a beginning, middle and end. By applying this universal principle to the art of sequencing (*vinyāsa krama*), an *āsana* practice is made more effective and efficient.

Sequencing creates the blueprint for a practice and consists of three stages:

- preparation for the goal posture (*pūrvāṅga*)
- arriving at the goal (*pradhānāṅga*)
- creating a smooth transition to the next activity (*uttaraṅga*)

Vinyāsa krama takes into account the activities we engage in before and after each practice. Although this chapter focuses on *āsana*, proper sequencing is a principle we also apply when designing practices for *prāṇāyāma* and meditation.

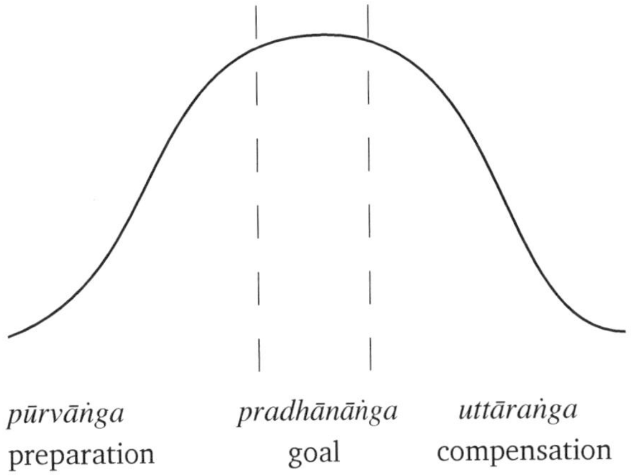

Stage 1: Preparation *(pūrvāṅga)*

If we fry garlic in a pan and then use it to make pancakes, our pancakes will taste like garlic unless we clean out the pan in-between. Simply put, *āsana* is a powerful tool for cleaning out the pan. A properly sequenced practice can eliminate the residue from our previous activity and prepare us to engage in our next pursuit with a fresh perspective.

The *pūrvāṅga* stage is usually the longest part of the practice, as it requires the most planning and consideration. First, we must decide the aim of the practice. Next, we carefully choose and sequence the poses which will prepare the body, breath and mind to reach the goal. These postures must be easier than the goal as well as similar in form and function.

Stage 2: Goal *Āsana (pradhānāṅga)*

The *pradhānāṅga* phase is the arrival at the goal posture. Here, all the components of preparation now enable us to achieve the *āsana* while maintaining the qualities of stability, comfort and long, smooth breathing.

Stage 3: Compensation/Completion *(uttāraṅga)*

Once we have achieved the goal pose, we must compensate and restore balance to our body, breath and mind. This stage also creates a smooth transition to our next activity, which could be *prāṇāyāma*, meditation, chanting or merely resuming our daily routine.

Methodology of Sequencing *Āsana*: The Six Guidelines

Incorporating the concepts from the previous chapter, here are six guidelines for designing a practice which is safe, elegant and efficient:

- Verify the ability to comfortably perform the reference posture for the goal pose.
- Begin with an easy, symmetrical posture in the appropriate orientation.
- Choose only *āsanas* that are simpler than the goal.
- Perform appropriate counterposes throughout.
- Rest as needed, especially between postures and before changing orientations.
- Finish with one or more counterposes to compensate and prepare for a final resting position, *prāṇāyāma* and/or meditation.

These guidelines for *āsana* practice help us set reasonable goals and logically sequence the steps to achieve them.

Three Practices

We will now present three different practices. Each one is sequenced to accomplish a specific goal. They are designed to:

- develop the ability to perform a specific *āsana*.
- create a desired energetic effect.
- achieve a specific, health-related benefit.

Note: In the following three practices, the numbers in the square box represent the order of the poses in the practice. The arrows indicate the direction of movement with the corresponding breath. We have also denoted the number of repetitions (3x = 3 times) and the length of the stay (stay 3 br = stay for three breaths).

The Aim of Practice 1: To Develop the Ability to Perform a Specific *Āsana*

First, choose a goal posture you would like to achieve. For this practice, we have chosen a seated, asymmetrical forward bend, *jānuśīrṣāsana*.

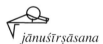

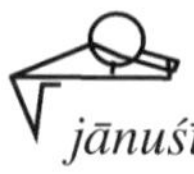
jānuśīrṣāsana

Next, verify that the reference posture (sitting on the floor) can be performed.

Because this forward bend is performed with one leg straight and one knee on the floor, we need to pick *āsana* that will stretch the back and the legs while opening the hips.

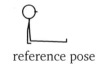

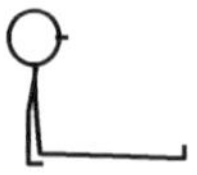
reference pose

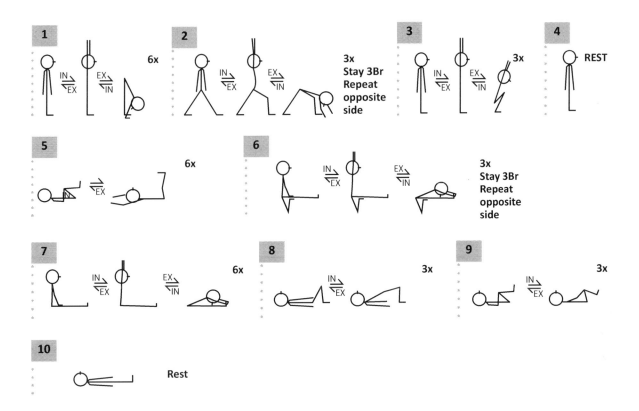

WHY WE DID WHAT WE DID:

PŪRVĀṄGA

1. In keeping with the classical order of orientation, we started with standing postures. For our first pose we chose *uttānāsana*, a symmetrical forward bend. It is in the same classification as the goal pose and stretches and strengthens the back.

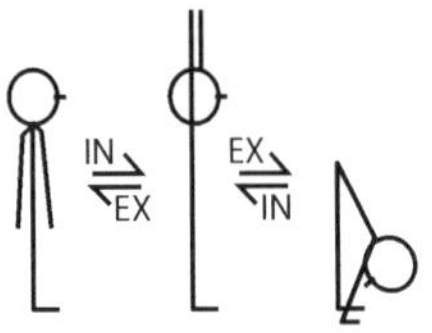

2. We selected the asymmetrical *vinyāsa krama* of a backbend (*vīrabhadrāsana*) to a forward bend (*pārśva uttānāsana*) because of its efficiency. *Vīrabadhrāsana* stretches the hips, while *pārśva uttānāsana* stretches the back and the back of the leg.

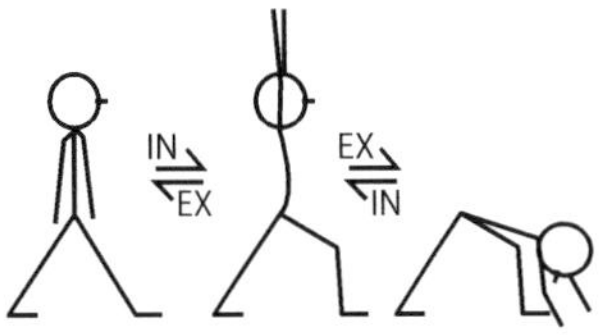

3. For a counterpose, we used *utkaṭāsana*, a symmetrical forward bend in the same orientation. Done dynamically, it realigns the body and relieves any stress from the previous postures. In addition, this pose stretches the ankles and adds greater flexibility to the hips.

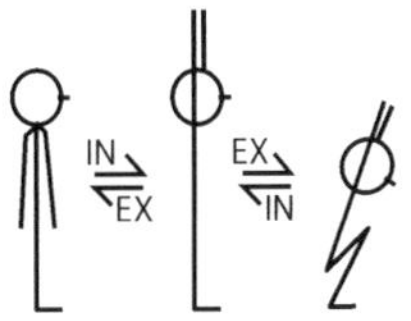

4. We rested in *samasthiti*, the same orientation (standing). This allows the body to recover, the breath to return to normal, and an opportunity to notice the effects of the previous postures.

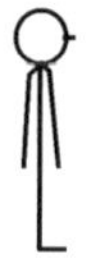

5. We moved to the next orientation, lying on the back. Here we performed *apānāsana* to *ūrdhva prasārita pādāsana*, a symmetrical *vinyāsa* that stretches the spine and the back of the legs while adding flexibility to the shoulders.

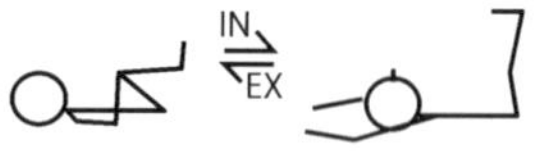

PRADHĀNĀṄGA

6. Having taken the steps to fully prepare the body, we were then able to perform *jānuśīrṣāsana* (the goal pose), both dynamically and statically, with ease.

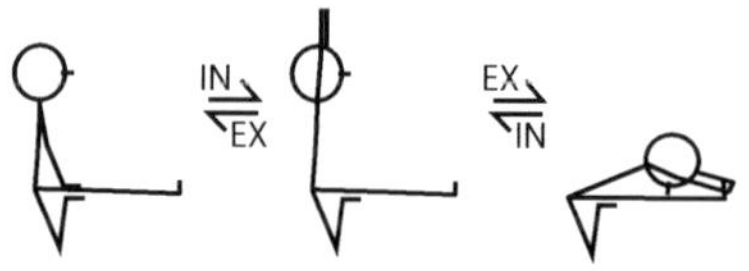

UTTARĀṄGA

7. Next, we performed *paścimatānāsana*, a symmetrical forward bend in the same orientation, which acts as a counterpose and realigns the body.

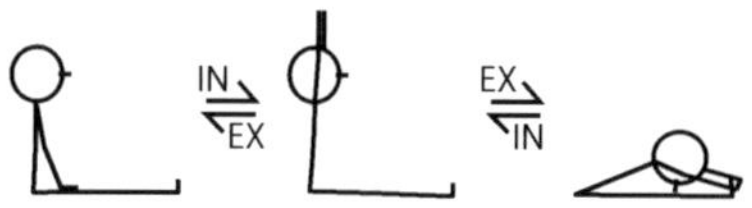

8. Transitioning to the supine orientation, we performed *dvipādapīṭham*. This backbend serves as a counterpose for the previous forward bends and provides a gentle stretch to the front of the body.

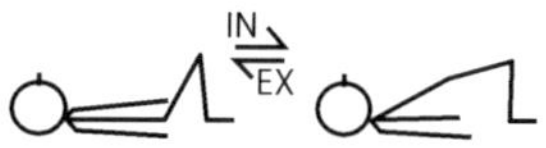

9. This final symmetrical forward bend, *apānāsana*, is a counterpose to the previous backbend. This provided an easy stretch to the lower back and moved us toward relaxation.

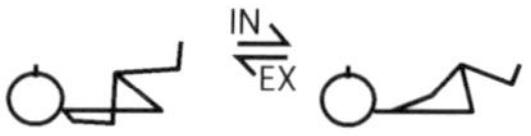

10. *Śavāsana* gave the body, breath and mind the opportunity to rest, integrate and savor the effects of the practice.

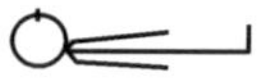

The Aim of Practice 2: To Achieve a Specific Energetic Effect

In this *bṛṁhaṇa* practice, we use dynamic postures to promote internal heat and increase energy. As backbends are more heating, we have chosen *bhujaṅgāsana* as the goal pose. We use several easier backbends to slowly build heat and prepare the body.

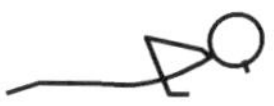

bhujaṅgāsana

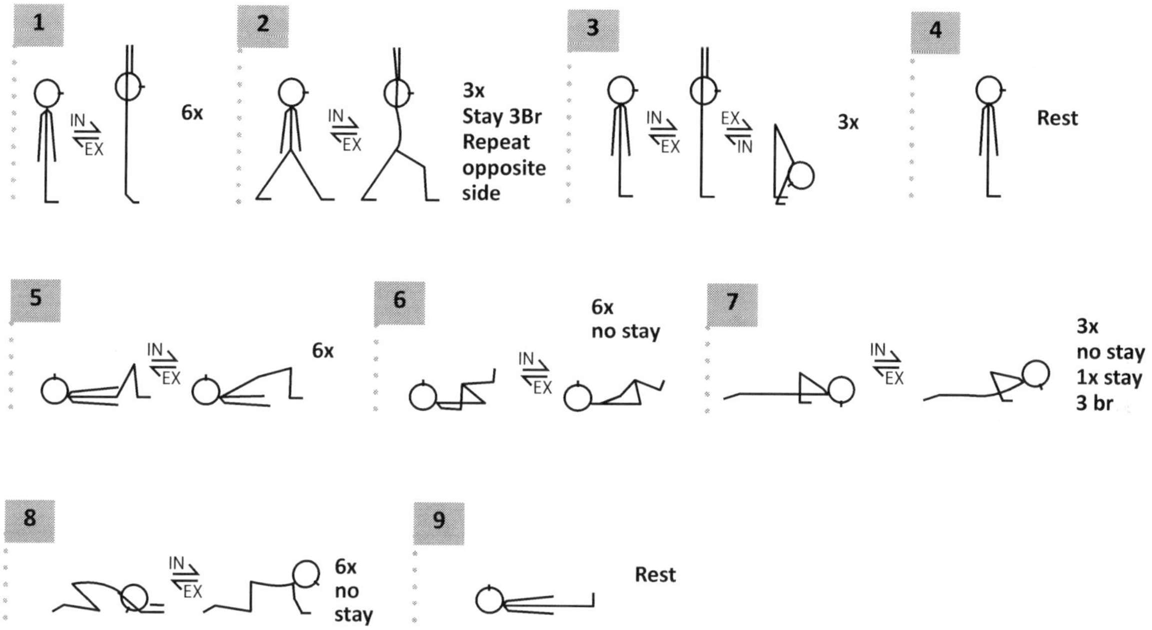

WHY WE DID WHAT WE DID:

PŪRVĀṄGA

1. In keeping with T. Krishnamacharya's order of orientation, we started with standing postures. We began with *tāḍāsana*, a symmetrical backbend. The combination of a moderate back arch done dynamically, along with the exertion of raising the heels and balancing, begins the heating effect.

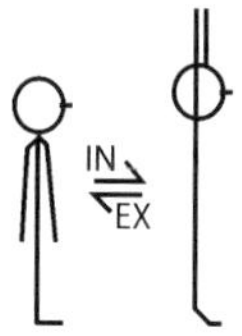

2. Next, came *vīrabhadrāsana*, an asymmetrical backbend. Also done dynamically, this pose expands the front of the body and works the large muscles of the legs, increasing the *bṛṁhaṇa* effect.

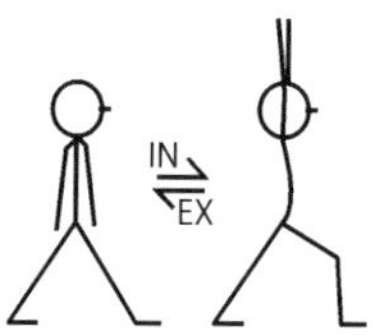

3. To counterpose, we chose *uttānāsana*, a symmetrical forward bend in the same orientation, done dynamically to stretch the back and legs.

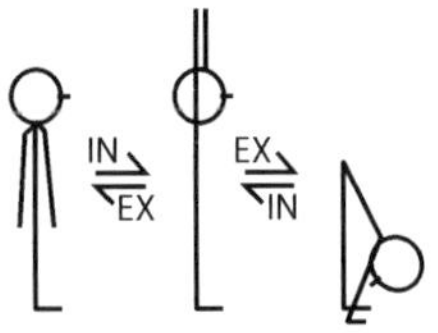

4. We rested in *samasthiti*, the reference pose for the standing orientation. This allows the body to recover and the breath to return to normal. It also provides an opportunity to observe the effects of the previous postures.

5. Then we moved to the next orientation, lying on the back, and performed *dvipādapīṭham* dynamically. This pose arches the back and expands the chest, creating more heat and preparing us for the goal posture.

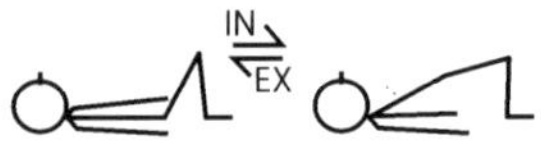

6. For a counterpose, we chose *apānāsana*, a forward bend in the same orientation, done dynamically. This stretches the lower back and brings the spine back to neutral.

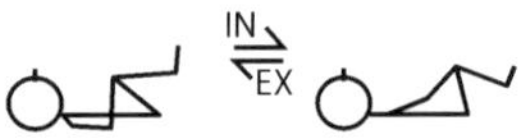

PRADHĀNĀṄGA

7. Having prepared and warmed the body appropriately, we were able to achieve the goal pose, *bhujaṅgāsana*. We first performed this *āsana* dynamically, then statically to achieve the desired energetic effect.

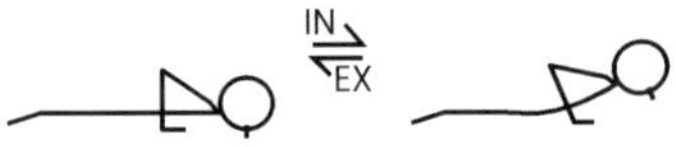

UTTARĀṄGA

8. Finally we moved in and out of *cakravākāsana,* to relieve any stress in the back and to maintain the *bṛṁhaṇa* effect.

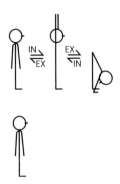

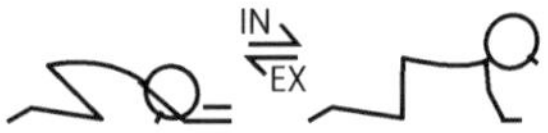

9. *Śavāsana* provides the body, breath and mind the opportunity to rest, integrate and savor the effects of the practice.

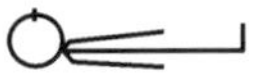

The Aim of Practice 3: To Achieve a Health-Related Benefit

In this practice, the health related benefit we are trying to achieve is increasing back strength. The strategy we have chosen is to alternate between forward bends and backbends done both dynamically and statically.

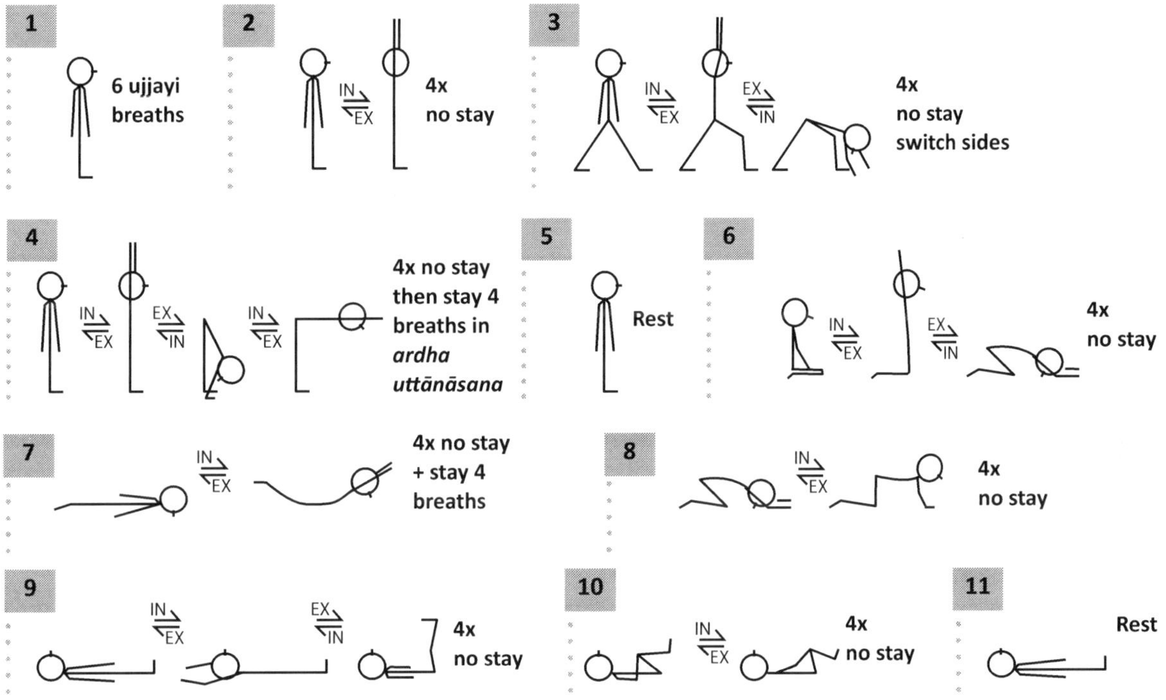

WHY WE DID WHAT WE DID:

PŪRVĀṄGA

1. Once again, we started with standing postures. For our first pose, we chose *samasthiti* to establish *ujjāyī* breathing.

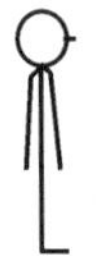

2. We raised and lowered the arms in *samasthiti* to coordinate breath with movement.

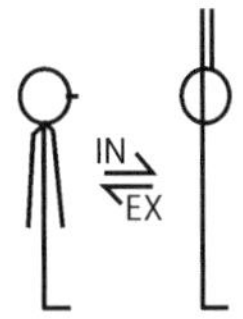

3. For efficiency, we linked the backbend (*vīrabhadrāsana*) with a forward bend (*pārśva uttānāsana*). *Vīrabhadrāsana* opens the chest and stretches the hips. Moving up from *pārśva uttānāsana* strengthens the back. This combination is a preparation for a stay in the next posture.

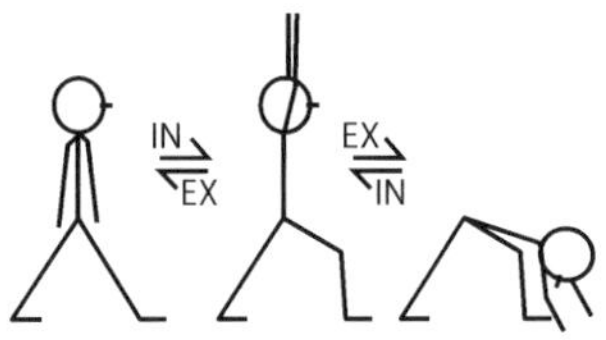

4. Next, we combined *uttānāsana* (a symmetrical forward bend) with *ardha uttānāsana* (a backbend). This *vinyāsa* serves as both a counterpose (*uttānāsana*) and another back-strengthening posture (*ardha uttānāsana*).

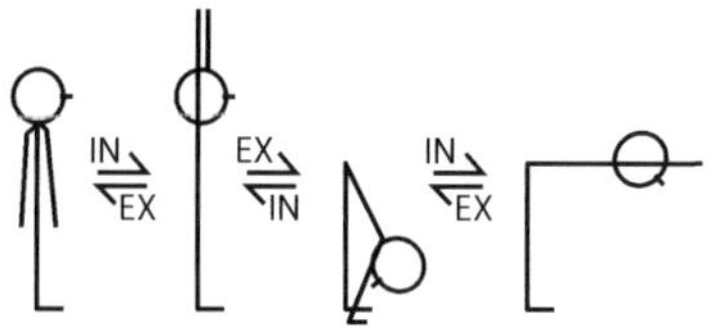

5. We rested in *samasthiti*, the standing reference pose. This allows the body to recover, the breath to return to normal, and gives us an opportunity to observe the effects of the previous postures.

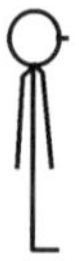

PRADHĀNĀṄGA

6. We chose our next posture (*vajrāsana*) to act as a transition to the kneeling orientation. Done dynamically, the forward bend stretches the back on the way down and strengthens it coming back up.

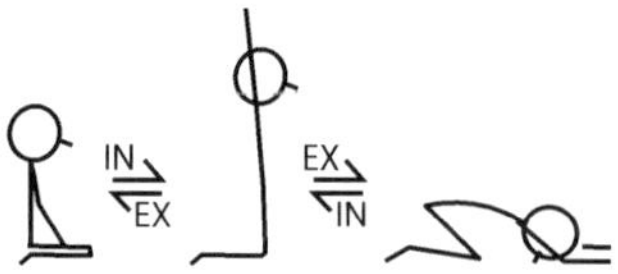

7. Moving to the next orientation, prone (lying on our stomach), we performed an intense backbend, *śalabhāsana*, to contract and further strengthen the back. We stayed in the pose for several breaths to increase the effect.

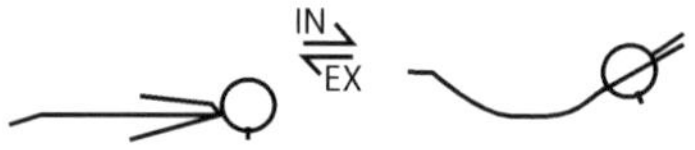

8. To counterpose and relax the back, we chose *cakravākāsana*, done dynamically.

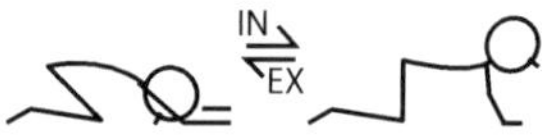

9. Moving to the supine position (lying on the back), we did *ūrdhva prasāritapādāsana* to support and strengthen the low back while working the abdominal muscles.

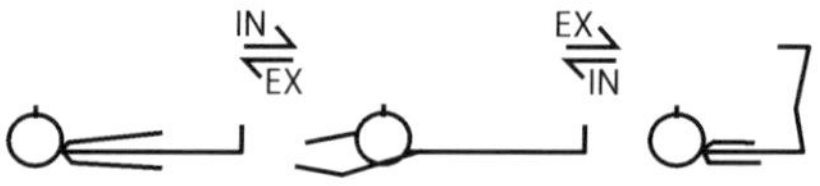

UTTARĀṄGA

10. For a final counterpose, we chose *apānāsana*, a forward bend in the same orientation, to relax the lower back.

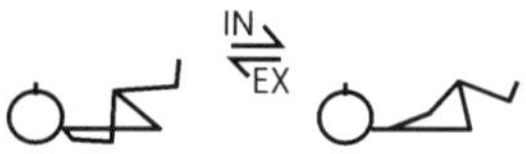

11. *Śavāsana* provided the body, breath and mind the opportunity to rest and integrate the effects of the practice.

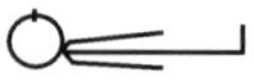

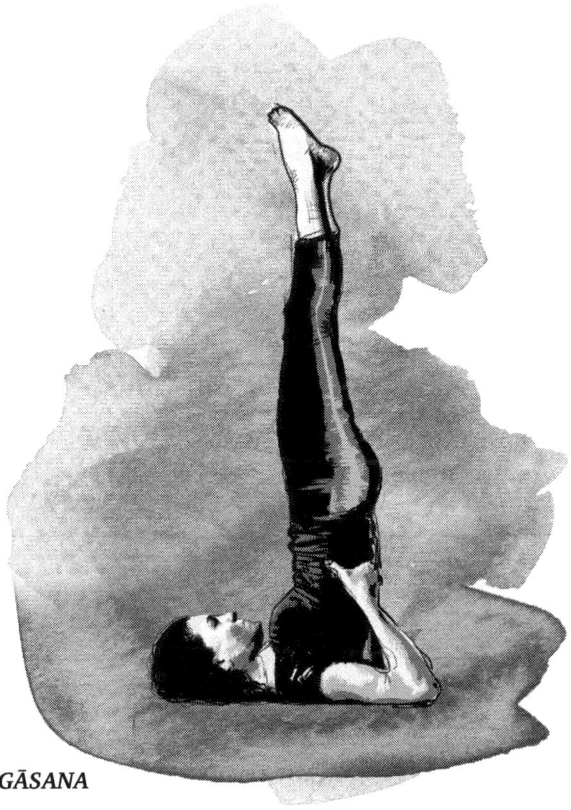

SARVAṄGĀSANA

Using Milestones to Plan for a Goal Posture over Time

A milestone is a significant point or benchmark in development. In sequencing, certain postures serve as milestones on our way to achieving a goal pose by verifying the specific physical requirements needed to accomplish that goal posture. For example, if your goal is to perform *śalabhāsana*, a pose that requires significant back strength, then you must first be able to achieve a milestone such as *bhujaṅgāsana*, an easier backbend.

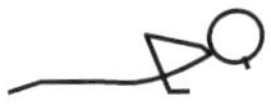

bhujaṅgāsana

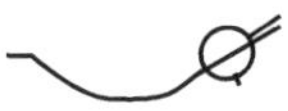

śalabhāsana

In the very process of trying to reach the goal pose, many things may change, including our reasons for wanting to achieve it. In practicing *Yoga*, the lessons learned on the journey often prove to be more beneficial than the destination itself.

The following three practices illustrate such a journey leading to a final goal, shoulderstand (*sarvaṅgāsana*). Along the way, specific milestones will prepare you and verify your ability to achieve this pose. In the first practice, the milestone is bridge pose (*dvipādapīṭham*), which introduces the *viparīta* (inversion) effect, while verifying the flexibility and strength of the neck and shoulders. Once you are able stay in bridge pose comfortably for 10 *ujjāyī* breaths, you can progress to the next practice.

In the second practice, the milestone is half shoulderstand (*viparītakaraṇī*). This inversion verifies the strength in the abdomen and back, as well as the flexibility in the hips, legs and spine needed for full shoulderstand (*sarvaṅgāsana*). When you are able to comfortably sustain a half shoulderstand for 10 *ujjāyī* breaths, you are ready for the goal pose, *sarvaṅgāsana*, in practice three.

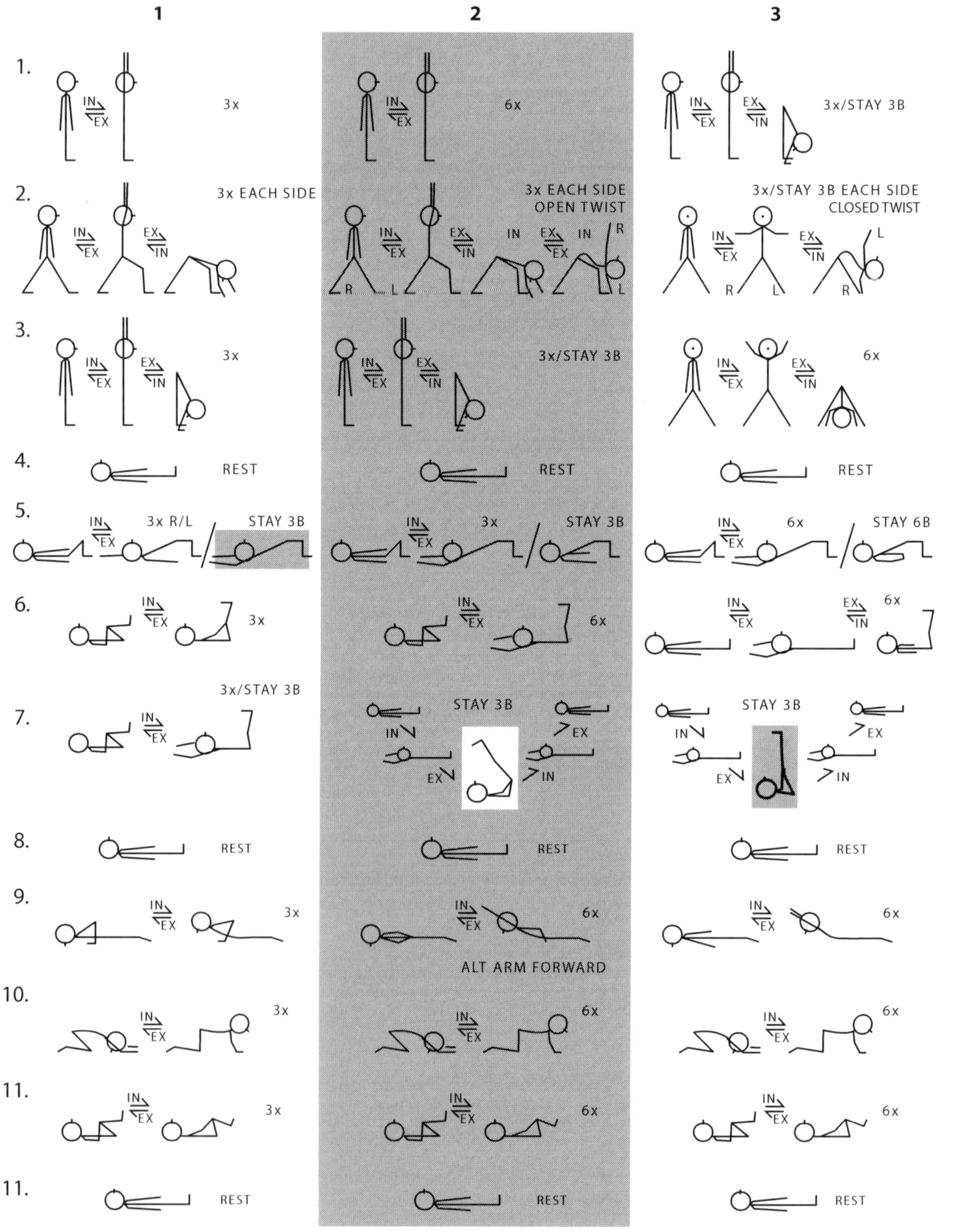

To Sum Up:

- *Vinyāsa krama* refers to:

  logical steps taken to perform each *āsana*.

  the correct arrangement of postures to achieve a goal within a single practice.

  planning a series of practices over time to achieve a specific goal.

- There are three stages to sequencing:

  1. preparation – *pūrvāṅga*
  2. goal – *pradhānāṅga*
  3. compensation/completion – *uttāraṅga*

- There are six guidelines for designing a practice which is safe, effective and efficient:

  1. verify the ability to comfortably perform the reference posture for the goal pose.
  2. begin with an easy, symmetrical posture in the appropriate orientation.
  3. choose only *āsanas* that are simpler than the goal.
  4. perform appropriate counterposes throughout.
  5. rest as needed, especially between postures and before changing orientations.
  6. finish with one or more counterposes to compensate and prepare for a final resting position, *prāṇāyāma* and/or meditation.

- Milestone postures help us plan a practice to achieve a goal over time.

CHAPTER 16

Sequencing, Part III: Adapting *Āsana* to the Individual

Constant change is an undeniable fact of life. Nowhere is this more evident than in our physical bodies. To paraphrase *Yoga* master T.K.V. Desikachar, for *Yoga* practice to be effective, it must be adapted to the individual, rather than the individual needing to adapt to the practice. The skillful modification of postures preserves the function of classical *āsana,* while respecting the individual's ever-changing needs and life conditions.

In order for *āsana* to continue to serve us over time, we must shift our focus from the idealized picture of what a pose should look like, its form, to the actual purpose of the posture, its function. This emphasis of function over form is the basis for all adaptation/modification.

Chris's story:

Over the years I have had many people approach me with an interest in *Yoga*. Often their desire was overshadowed by the fear that their lack of flexibility would prevent them from participating in a class.

Recently, I had a new student in a group class named Frank. He complained he was so stiff that he couldn't do *Yoga* postures like the ones he had seen. When bending over he could hardly touch his knees, let alone reach the floor, as in the classical forward bend. I explained that the form of the pose mattered less than its function, which was for him to feel a comfortable stretch in his back. I taught him to bend his knees and bring his hands to his shins. I pointed out that this modification would help him to achieve the same benefits as those enjoyed by students who could easily touch the floor. By the end of the class, his back felt better and he was filled with hope. Four years later, Frank's back is much stronger and he can now touch his ankles.

Modifications

The appropriate use of modifications in practice is part of a long-term process that slowly builds strength, flexibility and stamina. Ideally, there is a progression towards the classical pose (although we may never arrive), while respecting the needs and limitations of the individual. When we adapt an *āsana*, we change the form of the posture to make it easier while maintaining its function. Chris's student, Frank, was able to experience a stretch in his back even though the posture looked different than the classical form. By beginning with the modified posture, Frank learned to accept and work with his current limitations. As he moved toward the ideal posture, he began to cultivate patience and perseverance. Over time, his steady progression helped him develop confidence and optimism.

Techniques

In chapter 12, we explained how the spine's movement in all five directions determines the posture's function and must be the central focus of all *āsana*. To maintain the function of the pose, we sometimes need to change the position of the arms and legs. The following illustrations represent the classic form followed by some modifications.

Arm Modifications

As most postures involve moving the arms, let's start with some simple arm modifications. From left to right, the postures begin with the classical form and become easier. These can be used in any posture or orientation (standing, supine, kneeling, prone) that applies:

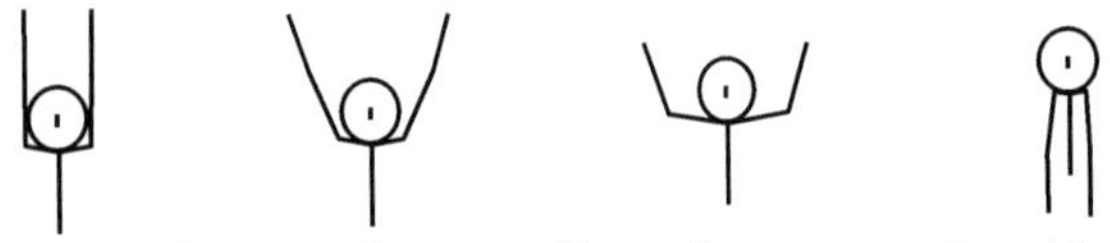

classical wide elbows bent arms by side

In classical postures, the arms are extended straight overhead, aligned with the ears. The shoulders are down and the chest is open, allowing for a deep inhale. If your shoulders rise toward the ears or move forward when you lift your arms, then a modification is needed.

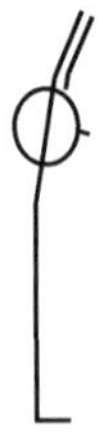

As a rule, choose the arm position closest to the classical posture that best facilitates the extension of your spine and expansion of your chest. Whichever position you choose, you must be able to perform it with both stability and comfort in the body, breath and mind.

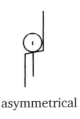

asymmetrical

Another option is raising the arms asymmetrically (one at a time). This is a helpful modification for those who lack the strength or flexibility to raise both arms.

Leg Modifications

The legs serve as the foundation for all standing postures. Practitioners with tight hamstrings, a stiff back, tight hips or poor balance should bend the knees and/or widen the legs as needed.

Here are some examples in three orientations (standing, seated and supine):

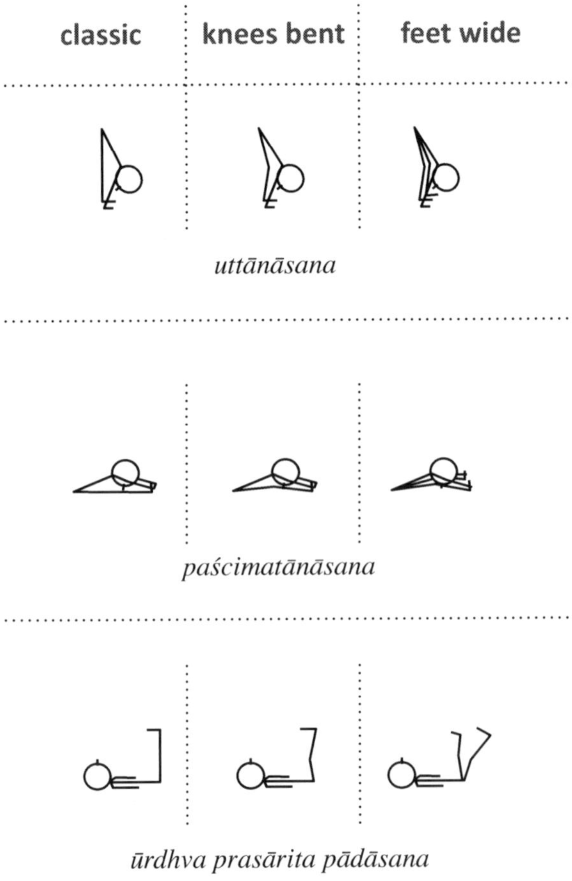

Range of Movement

If you lack the strength or flexibility to perform the classic posture, the modification would be to go only as far into the pose as you comfortably can.

classic | modified

uttānāsana

vajrāsana

Going partway into the pose ensures our comfort, preserves the function of the *āsana* and increases our range of movement over time.

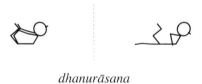

dhanurāsana

Use of props

Rather than using *Yoga* props to force the body into the ideal form of the pose, ordinary household items (chairs, walls and cushions) can be used as props to achieve the posture's function while maintaining the feeling of *sthira/sukha*.

In any practice, there is a logical sequence to knowing when and how to perform a posture with a modification or a prop to achieve the function of the pose.

- First try the classical pose.
- Modify the posture as needed.
- Try using an appropriate prop.
- Consider a different pose.

The use of props should always provide support rather than force, promote an inward focus and allow us to experience the practice without distraction.

Following are some examples of using ordinary props:

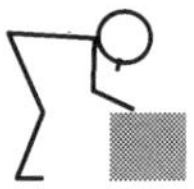

uttānāsana
standing to chair

uttānāsana
forward bend seated on chair

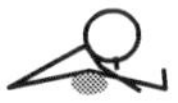

paścimatānāsana
seated with a cushion under knees

tāḍāsana
with one arm

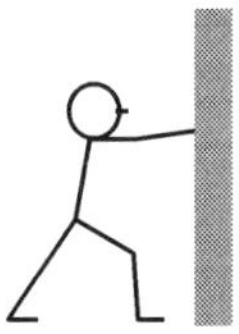

virabhradhrāsana
to wall

śavāsana
with a cushion under knees

Applications

Following are the three practices from chapter 15 using modifications to accommodate limitations and help achieve the same goals and benefits of the practices.

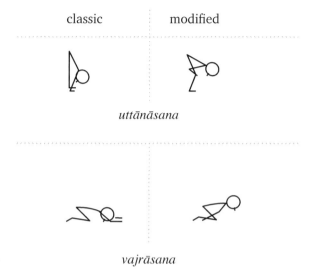

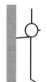

The Aim of Practice 1, with Modifications: To Develop the Ability to Perform a Specific *Āsana*

Our goal pose for Practice 1 is a modified version of *jānuśīrṣāsana*, a seated, asymmetrical forward bend.

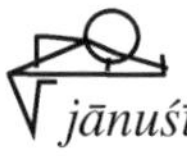

jānuśīrṣāsana

Just as in the classic posture, we still need to verify that the reference posture (sitting on the floor) can be performed.

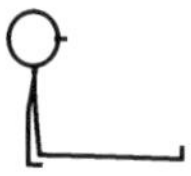

reference posture

This practice will be modified for someone with stiff shoulders or a tight upper back.

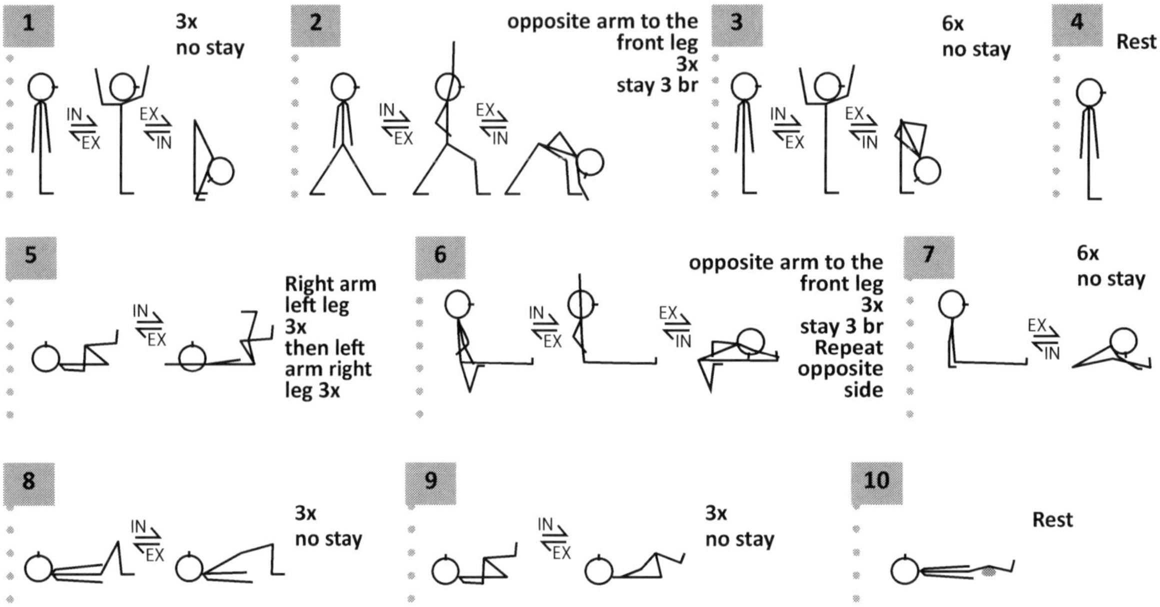

WHY WE DID WHAT WE DID:

PŪRVĀṄGA

1. We started in the standing orientation. To accommodate the tight upper back and stiff shoulders, we performed *uttānāsana* with the arms bent.

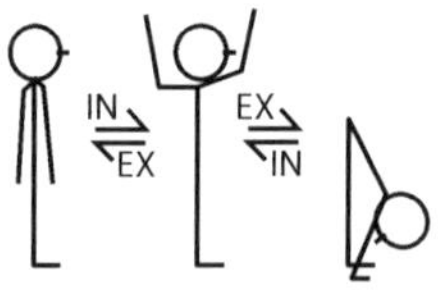

2. Next, we modified the asymmetrical *vinyāsa krama* of a backbend (*vīrabhadrāsana*) to a forward bend (*pārśva uttānāsana*) by placing the same arm as the front leg on the small of the back and performed the entire *vinyāsa* with the other arm. This lightens the load on the back. In addition, we bent the front leg as we folded forward to feel the back stretch and accommodate tightness in the hamstrings.

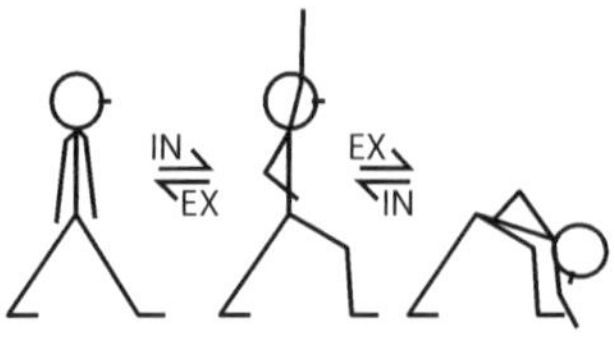

3. We modified the counterpose, *uttānāsana*, by sweeping the arms out to the side (bending the arms if needed), bringing them to the small of the back as we bent forward. This reduces any stress in the neck and shoulders while stretching the back.

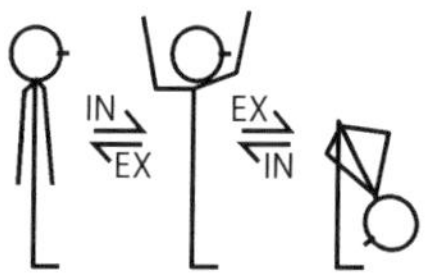

4. We rested in *samasthiti*, the same orientation, (standing).

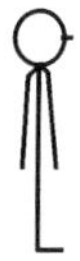

5. Lying on the back in *apānāsana*, we modified *ūrdhva prasārita pādāsana* by making it asymmetrical. Alternately raising one arm and the opposite leg ensures less stress on the shoulders and hamstrings.

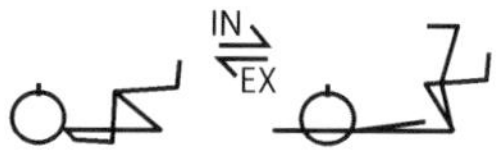

PRADHĀNĀṄGA

6. To account for any tightness in the shoulders, back and legs, we modified the goal pose, *jānuśīrṣāsana*, by repeating the adaptations from number 2.

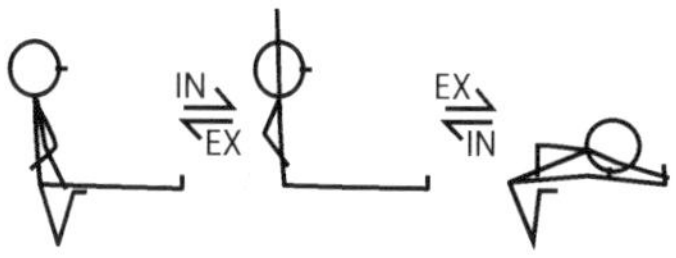

UTTARĀṄGA

7. We modified the counterpose, *paścimatānāsana*, by sliding our hands down the legs to reduce the stress in the back. We bent the knees to address the tightness in the hamstrings.

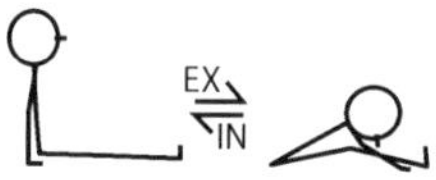

8. Not modified.

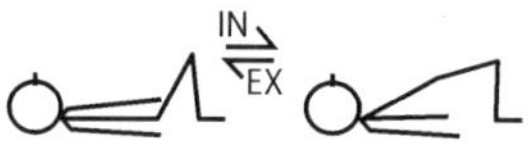

9. Not modified.

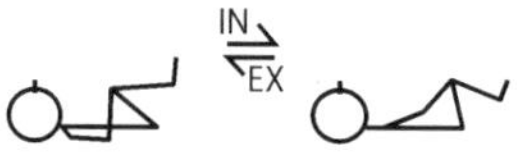

10. To modify *śavāsana*, we placed a pillow or rolled blanket under the knees. This reduces the curve in the lower back, making it more comfortable for the back, neck and shoulders.

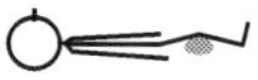

The Aim of Practice 2, with Modifications: To Achieve a Specific Energetic Effect

In this modified *bṛṁhaṇa* practice, we will modify the postures for someone with low energy or stooped shoulders and rounded upper back. A modified *bhujaṅgāsana* is the goal pose.

modified *bhujaṅgāsana*

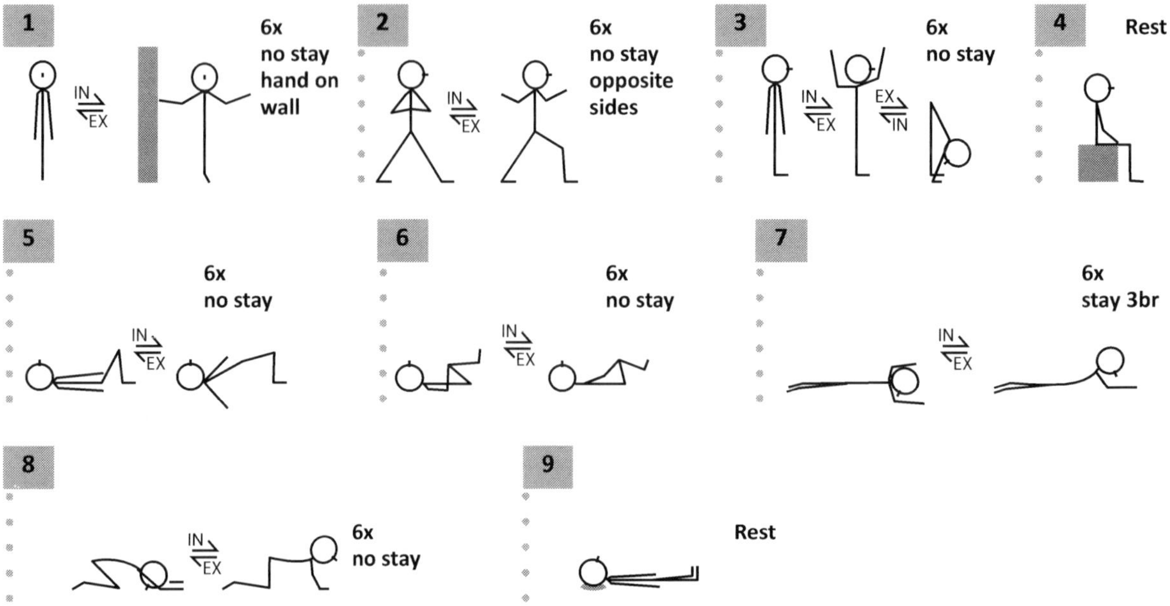

WHY WE DID WHAT WE DID:

PŪRVĀṄGA

1. We began with a modified *tāḍāsana*. To help with balance, we placed one hand on a wall about shoulder height and came up on the toes while raising the other arm halfway to accommodate the rounded upper back.
2. For modified *vīrabhadrāsana*, we started with our hands resting on the chest. We came into the pose opening the bent arms out to the side to help expand the chest and flatten the upper back.
3. Our modified counterpose, *uttānāsana*, was done with arms wide to keep the upper back flat.
4. To accommodate the low energy, we rested in *samasthiti* in a chair.

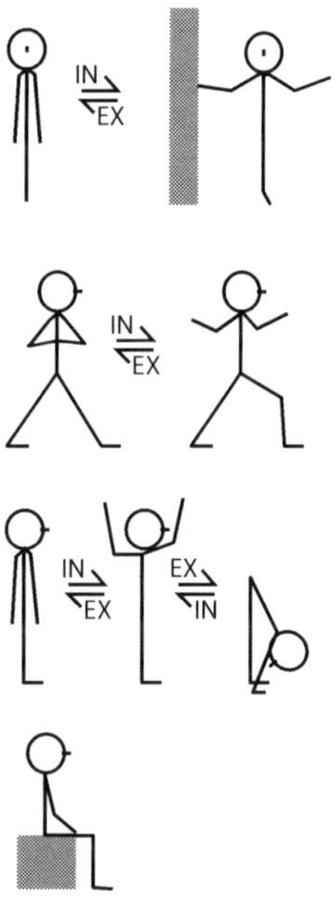

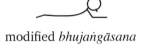

5. Lying on the back, we performed *dvipādapīṭham* with arms on the floor, shoulder height and palms up. This expands the chest and prepares us for the goal pose.

6. *Apānāsana* is not modified.

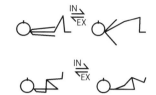

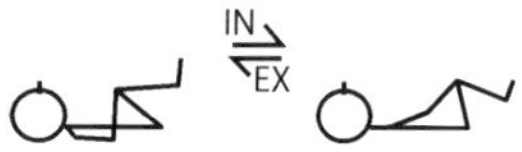

PRADHĀNĀṄGA

7. To address the stooped shoulders and low energy we modified the goal pose *bhujaṅgāsana* by keeping the elbows on the floor and lifting the chest partway.

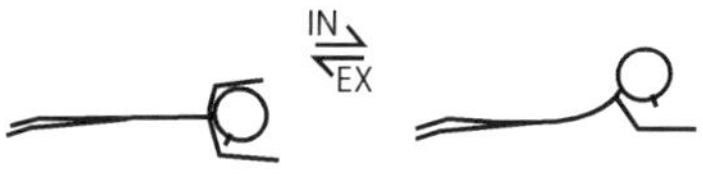

UTTARĀṄGA

8. The counterpose, *cakravākāsana*, is not modified.

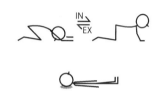

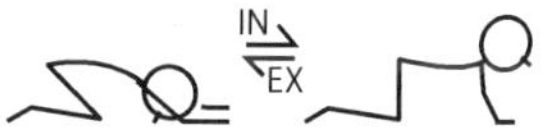

9. The final pose *śavāsana is* modified with a pillow to support the neck and shoulders.

The Aim of Practice 3, with Modifications: To Achieve a Health-Related Benefit

We modified this back-strengthening practice for a person with a sedentary lifestyle who lacks strength and flexibility. In order to strengthen the back, our goal is a modified *śalabhāsana*.

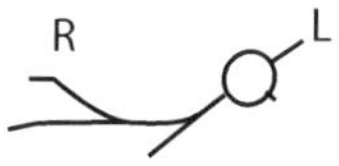

modified *śalabhāsana*

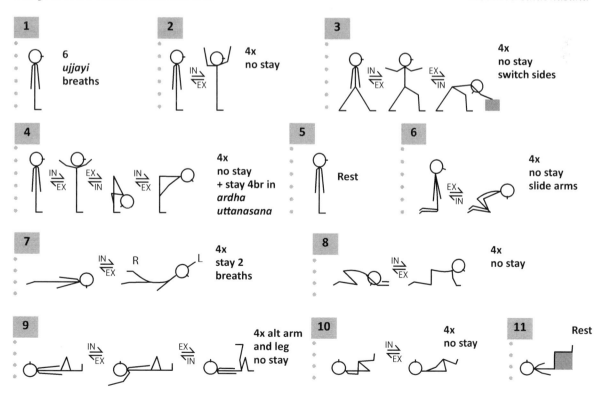

WHY WE DID WHAT WE DID:

PŪRVĀṄGA

1. We started standing in *samasthiti*.
2. We modified *samasthiti* by raising the arms halfway to accommodate the lack of strength in the arms and limited flexibility in the shoulders.
3. In this modified *vinyāsa*, we brought the arms wide in *vīrabhadrāsana* and used a chair in *pārśva uttānāsana* to accommodate the low energy and lack of flexibility.
4. We modified the next *vinyāsa* by widening the arms for the tight shoulders and bending the knees slightly in *uttānāsana* to respect the tight back and hamstrings. Next, we slid the hands partway up the legs into *ardha uttānāsana* to support with the weak back.
5. No modification in *samasthiti*.
6. In the modification of *vajrāsana*, we accounted for the lack of strength in the back by sliding the hands up and down the legs while moving in and out of the forward bend.

PRADHĀNĀṄGA

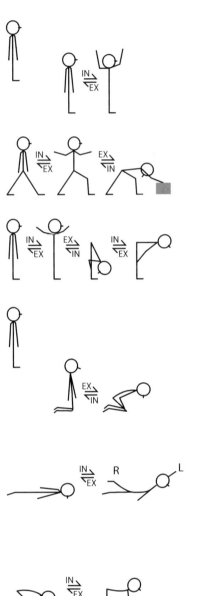

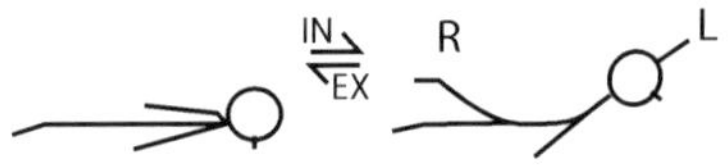

7. In our modified goal pose, *śalabhāsana*, we accommodated for all the limitations by simultaneously lifting the chest and one leg off the floor while sweeping the opposite arm forward.

UTTARĀṄGA

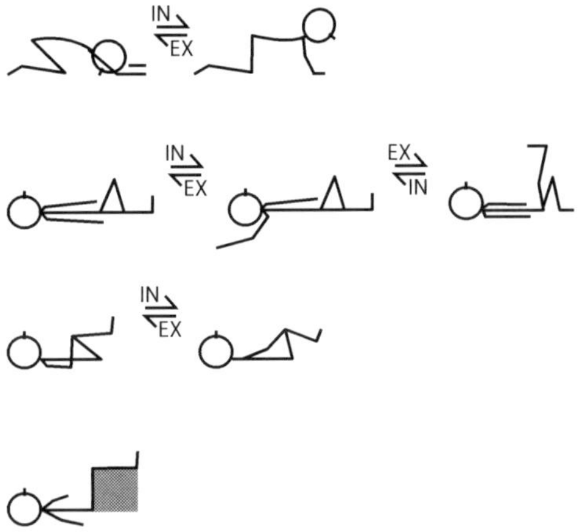

8. The counterpose *cakravākāsana* is not modified.
9. In the modified *ūrdhva prasārita pādāsana* we accommodated for the lack of strength in the back and flexibility in the legs by keeping one leg bent and raising only one arm.
10. The counterpose *apānāsana* is not modified.
11. *Śavāsana* is modified by elevating the bent legs and resting them on a chair. This takes the pressure off the low back, allowing for a deeper rest and recovery.

In the *Yoga Sūtras*, Patañjali teaches that all *Yoga* must be adapted to the individual. As these three practices illustrate, learning, implementing and ultimately mastering the art of modification insures that our *Yoga* will continue to serve us in the face of whatever changes we encounter in our lives.

To Sum Up:

- Just as life is constantly changing, we must change our practice over time.
- In *āsana*, we should prioritize function over form.
- We can preserve the function of *āsana* through modification.
- Modifications are accomplished by:
  1. changing the position of arms and legs
  2. varying the range of movement
  3. using simple props

CHAPTER 17

The Art of Conscious Breathing: *Prāṇāyāma*/The Fourth Limb

Although studies now validate the link between the breath and the mind, it was the ancient *yogis* who first used *prāṇāyāma* (conscious breathing techniques) to improve their physiological functioning as well as their mental and emotional states.

Prāṇāyāma, the Fourth Limb

Much like the electricity that powers our appliances, *prāṇa* is an invisible force that energizes the body and mind. The practice of *prāṇāyāma* extends and expands this life force. While *prāṇa* is not literally oxygen, the quality of our breathing is a measure of our *prāṇa*, as well as the link between our body and mind. When *prāṇa* is activated, the results are increased vitality and clearer communication, as well as improved digestion, elimination and circulation.

According to the *Prāṇa Vāyu* Model, the five primary manifestations of *prāṇa* are located in specific areas of the body and are responsible for various physiological functions.

Prāṇa vāyu, located in the chest, is responsible for respiration, specifically the inhale and all that we take in through our senses.

Apāna vāyu is located in the lower abdomen. It governs all downward movement, including elimination, menstruation and childbirth.

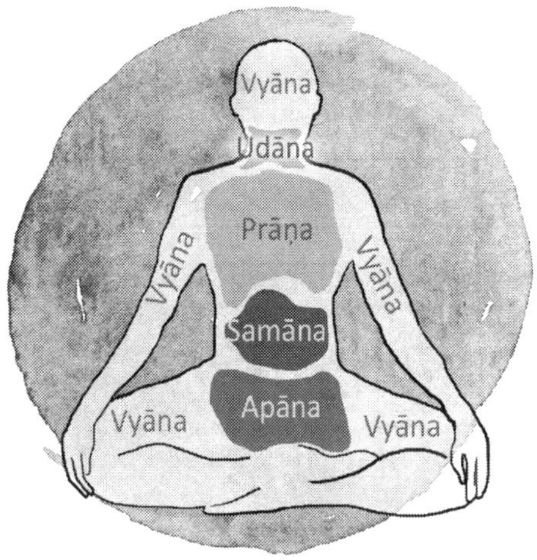

Samāna vāyu, located in the solar plexus, is responsible for the digestion and assimilation of food.

Udāna vāyu, located in the throat area, controls all upward movement including our exhale and vocal communication.

Finally, ***vyāna vāyu*** is responsible for circulating vitality throughout the body through the movement of oxygenated blood and nerve impulses.

By consciously focusing our attention on the breath we are able to activate and control our *prāṇa*. For this reason, over time, the continued practice of *prāṇāyāma* promotes optimal functioning of all five *vāyus*.

The Benefits of *Prāṇāyāma*

Along with helping us maintain optimal physiological functioning, *prāṇāyāma* also has many therapeutic applications.

In today's fast-paced world, short, shallow, stress-induced chest breathing is all too common, all too often, in all too many of us. This pattern engages the sympathetic nervous system, specifically the "fight or flight" response. Unlike our canine friends, who quickly shake off a surge of adrenaline, we humans accumulate and retain stress hormones in our system. As a result, we experience irregular heartbeat, indigestion, insomnia and a host of other stress-related conditions, all of which further distort our breathing and, as illustrated in the following story, our perception of reality.

Robert's Story:

While attending an out-of-town conference, I was awakened in my hotel room at 3 a.m. by a fire alarm and an urgent announcement over the loud speaker, "Grab what you need and evacuate the building immediately!" I bolted out of bed... gasping for breath...my chest heaving…my heart pounding... I had visions of jumping from my 13th floor window into a fireman's tiny net below. Using my best, albeit impaired, judgment under the circumstances, I grabbed the few things I deemed essential to my survival and ran into the hallway. As the door slammed and locked behind me, I looked down, still hyperventilating, and saw what I was clutching to my chest: a computer power cord, some dental floss and a sock. You know—the really important stuff.

Whether you're fleeing a burning building, called on the carpet by your boss or cut off by a bad driver, the resulting stress could lead to shallow breathing, raised blood pressure, a body flooded with adrenaline and a brain impaired by poor judgment.

In the practice of *prāṇāyāma*, we attempt to lengthen the breath, while consciously directing it to the lower third of the lungs. Because of the parasympathetic receptors located in this area, this method of breathing engages the "relaxation response." This antidote to the fight-or-flight response lowers our heart rate and reduces our blood pressure, thus improving the quality of our digestion and elimination. It also helps our mind become calmer, clearer and better prepared for meditation.

In order to deepen our understanding of the practice and benefits of *prāṇāyāma*, it is helpful to familiarize ourselves with the theory behind it as described in the ancient models. Let's begin by referring back to the energetic *Prāṇa/Agni/Mala* Model discussed in Part I.

Prāṇāyāma and the *Prāṇa/Agni/Mala* Model

The *Prāṇa/Agni/Mala* Model can be applied to both *āsana* and *prāṇāyāma*. In *āsana*, connecting the breath with movement strengthens the muscles of the torso and extends the spine. This creates space in the chest, which enables us to breathe more easily into the lower part of the lungs. It also increases the flow of oxygenated blood, nourishes the cells and relaxes the entire system.

Prāṇāyāma further activates *prāṇa*, ignites the *agni* (digestive fire) and draws it toward the *mala* (undigested experiences, food and toxins). In this model, excess *mala* contributes to mental agitation. By consciously extending the exhale, we move the *mala* closer to the *agni*, purifying the system and reducing distraction. In this way, the practice of *prāṇāyāma* helps prepare the mind for meditation.

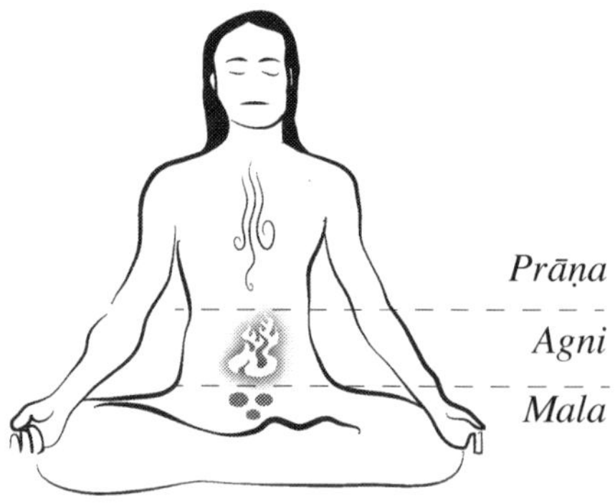

Prāṇāyāma and the *Nāḍīs*

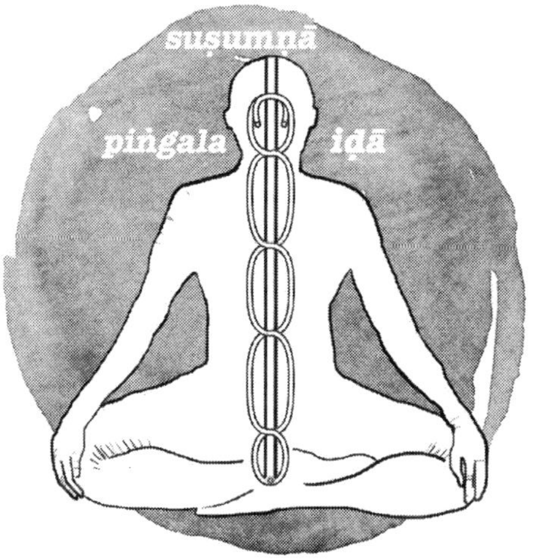

According to *Yoga* teachings, *prāṇa* flows through thousands of *nāḍīs*, or channels, in the human system. The three most important ones are located near the center of the body. *Iḍā* and *piṅgala*, the left and right channels crisscross the spine and terminate at the nostrils. *Suṣumṇā*, the central channel, originates at the base of the spine and carries *prāṇa* to the crown of the head. The purpose of all *prāṇāyāma* techniques is to direct *prāṇa* from the *iḍā* and *piṅgala nāḍīs* to the *suṣumṇā*. Increased *prāṇa* flowing through the *suṣumṇā nāḍī* is thought to improve all mental and physiological functions and create a more focused mind.

Prāṇāyāma and the *Yoga Sūtras*

Throughout the world, the *Yoga Sūtras* are considered the foundational text for the correct understanding of *prāṇāyāma*. According to Patañjali, *prāṇāyāma* is the most effective tool for linking the body and mind. It creates a powerful bridge between the gross external and, more subtle, internal worlds.

The *sutras*, defining *prāṇāyāma*, discuss the regulation of the four parts of the breath: the inhale, the exhale and the holds after each. However, *prāṇāyāma* is more than just controlling the breath. Because breathing is normally an unconscious process, the first step is to create an awareness of our own breathing patterns. With this awareness, we are then able to regulate the breath to create a desired effect.

Have you ever noticed whether you breathe through your nose or your mouth? When you take a breath does your chest expand, your belly move or both? Which is longer, your inhale or exhale? If you are like most of us, chances are you probably haven't paid much attention to these things.

To help increase our awareness and regulate the breath, Patañjali offers three components of practice: *deśa* (place), (*kāla*) time and *sāṃkhya* (duration).

Deśa

The first component, place or location(*deśa*), has several aspects:

- where we regulate the breath (the nostrils, tongue or throat)
- where we focus our attention (on concrete objects such as the heart or navel, or on abstract concepts such as compassion or gratitude)
- where we choose to practice (in a *Yoga* studio, on a mountaintop, in bed before sleep, etc.)

Kāla

The second component, time (*kāla*), refers to:

- the length of all four parts of the breath and their relationship to one another
- the time of day
- the season of the year
- the stage of life

Sāṃkhya

The third component, **duration** (*sāṃkhya*), addresses:

- the specific number of breaths in a given practice
- the length of time spent doing *prāṇāyāma*
- the frequency of practice

Patañjali states that when the four parts of the breath and the three components of practice are correctly combined, the result is breathing that is both long and smooth.

Common *Prāṇāyāma* Myths

Are you currently doing a *prāṇāyāma* practice? If not, you are not alone. Despite the proven benefits of *prāṇāyāma*, many *Yoga* students are unclear as to the proper method or even hesitant to approach this ancient practice. This is understandable, considering the subtle nature of *prāṇāyāma* and its diverse, often contradictory teachings. The many misperceptions and myths that have arisen around its practice have created confusion about the techniques and overshadowed the tremendous value of *prāṇāyāma*.

The prevailing myths concerning *prāṇāyāma* include:

- One must master all *āsana* before beginning the practice of *prāṇāyāma*.
- *Prāṇāyāma* practice is complex, difficult and boring.
- *Prāṇāyāma* is an esoteric practice requiring an exotic initiation.
- *Prāṇāyāma* can be dangerous and lead to disease or mental disorder.

To help distinguish these misconceptions from the proven truths about *prāṇāyāma*, we must first recognize certain minimum prerequisites that must be met before starting practice. In order to begin a *prāṇāyāma* practice, we should:

- have a clear intention and goal.
- practice on an empty stomach.
- set aside time for uninterrupted practice.
- perform appropriate *āsana* to prepare the body and mind.
- be able to maintain a comfortable, seated position and a straight spine (with support if needed).
- have the necessary attention span.

When you dispel the myths and meet the prerequisites for *prāṇāyāma*, you are ready to experience one of *Yoga*'s most subtle and effective tools. This powerful practice is highly effective in helping to achieve the clarity of mind that is *Yoga*'s ultimate goal.

To Sum Up:

- Most of us go through life with little or no awareness of our breathing.
- Conscious breathing techniques can improve our energy, health, attitude and behaviors.
- *Prāṇāyāma* extends and expands the life force (*prāṇa*) responsible for optimal functioning of all the systems of the body.
- In the *Prāṇa Vāyu* Model, there are five *vāyus* responsible for various physiological functions.
- *Prāṇāyāma* engages the parasympathetic nervous system, activates the relaxation response and prepares the practitioner for meditation.
- *Prāṇāyāma* is referenced in the *Prāṇa/Agni/Mala* and *Nāḍīs* Models and the *Yoga Sūtras*.
- The overall strategy in *prāṇāyāma* is to manipulate the four parts of the breath (inhale, exhale and pauses after each) with respect to place of focus, time and duration.
- *Prāṇāyāma* need not be boring or dangerous — in fact, it is one of *Yoga*'s most subtle and effective tools.

CHAPTER 18

Developing a *Prāṇāyāma* Practice

In the previous chapter, we explored the fundamental relationship between the breath, physical health and mental stability. While *āsana* is *Yoga*'s primary tool for refining and maintaining the physical body, *prāṇāyāma* is the tool for refining the breath. To quote the *Haṭha Yoga Pradīpikā*, "*chale vāte, chalaṁ cittaṁ*" or "as the breath goes, so the mind goes." In other words, the breath is not only an accurate gauge of our current psychological and emotional state, but can also serve as a powerful tool for changing them. Slow, deep breathing, cultivated by consistent *prāṇāyāma* practice, creates mental stability and is a prerequisite for meditation. Though the common perception is that better breathing means taking in a greater quantity of air, the true aim of *prāṇāyāma* is to change the quality of our breath and bring conscious attention to the breathing process. Patañjali refers to this improved quality as being both *dīrgha* (long) and *sūkṣma* (smooth).

In this chapter, we will discuss the best postures for practicing *prāṇāyāma*, the proper progression for developing the breath and the ways to integrate classical *mudrās* with various *prāṇāyāma* techniques.

There are two fundamental components of *prāṇāyāma*, ratio and technique. Ratio refers to the length of all four parts of the breath; inhale, hold after inhale, exhale, hold after exhale and their relationship to each another. We generally introduce ratio prior to techniques as it only requires the ability to valve the breath by constricting the throat (*ujjāyī*) and counting.

In the context of *prāṇāyāma*, techniques refer to the various methods for regulating or valving the flow of the breath through the nostrils, tongue and/or throat. *Mudrās* or hand gestures, are used in techniques which involve valving through the nostrils.

In addition to ratios and techniques, *pranayama* teaches us to consciously place our attention on expanding our chest on each inhale and contracting our abdomen on every exhale. This further lengthens the breath and keeps the spine erect.

A note of caution: Because each part of the breath (inhale, exhale and the holds after each) has the potential to either enhance or disturb the others, we must ensure that no part of the breath becomes uncomfortable.

Postures for *Prāṇāyāma*

There are several postures appropriate for the practice of *prāṇāyāma*. Below are choices that might work for you. Choose the most comfortable one that will allow you to keep your spine straight.

If sitting is not possible, try lying on your back.

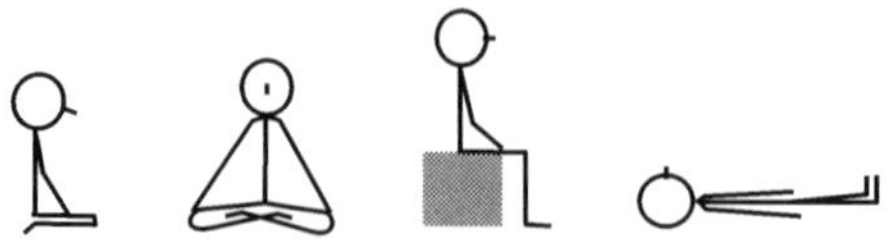

Note: Although lying on your back is effective for beginners learning *ujjāyī*, many *prāṇāyāma* techniques cannot be performed effectively in this position. In addition, performing *prāṇāyāma* lying on the back might cause you to become distracted and drowsy.

Mudrās for *Prāṇāyāma*

In addition to the correct postures, specific *prāṇāyāma* techniques also employ various *mudrās*. *Mudrās* are hand positions, often with symbolic meanings, which direct our physical energy and mental attention in a particular direction. They are created by placing the fingers together and/or placing the hands on a specific part of the body. Though there are many possible *mudrās*, let's examine the two that we commonly use in *prāṇāyāma*, *cin mudrā* and *mṛgi mudrā*.

Cin Mudrā

This is the standard hand position for most *prāṇāyāma* techniques. Sit with both hands resting on your knees, palms facing upward. With each hand, bring the tip of the index finger and thumb together to form a circle. The continuous contact between your thumbs and fingers creates a sense of a closed energy circuit and adds an additional point of focus for vour attention.

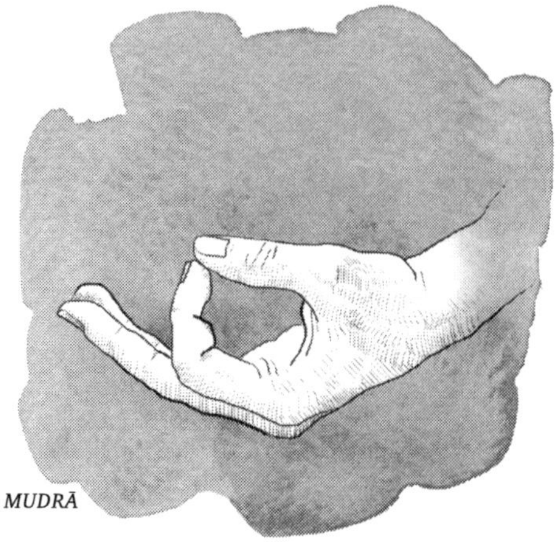

CIN MUDRĀ

Mṛgi Mudrā

This *mudrā* is used for all nostril techniques. Begin in a seated position with your hands resting on your knees, palms facing upward. Place your left hand in *cin mudrā*. With your right hand make a fist and extend the pinkie, ring finger and thumb. If possible, keep the pinkie and ring fingers touching. In the technique section, we will learn how to use this *mudrā* in *prāṇāyāma*.

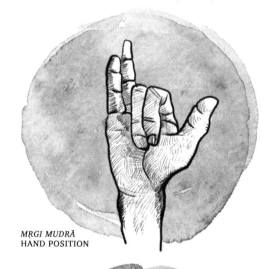

MṚGI MUDRĀ
HAND POSITION

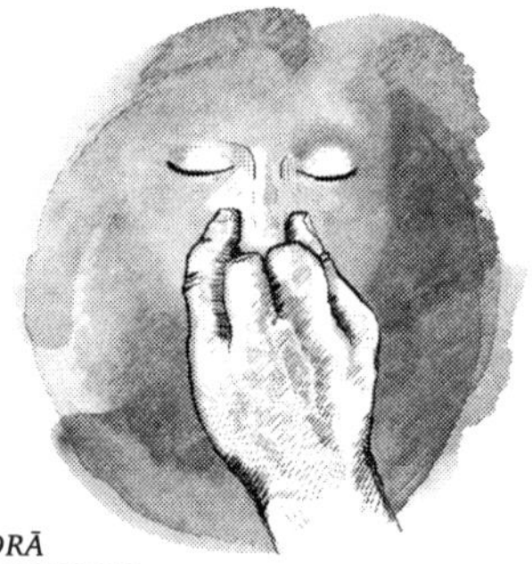

MṚGI MUDRĀ
NOSTRIL POSITION

Practices for Developing the Breath

The process of applying the above tools will be explained in the following practices. These practices are progressive, illustrating precisely where to begin and how to evolve over time. We suggest you take as much time as needed to learn each practice, as well as to experience and integrate its benefits, before moving on to the next. If you experience any discomfort such as feeling out of breath or increased heart rate, stop and let the breath return to normal, then begin again, possibly with less-challenging lengths. It is important never to force the breath and maintain an even, smooth, comfortable range.

The following practices all consist of 12 breaths. We have found that this is the minimum number of breaths needed to experience the effects of *prāṇāyāma*.

Note: Technically, a pause is 2 seconds or less and a hold is 3 seconds or more. A hold can be any desired length, providing it creates no tension, agitation or discomfort.

Practice 1: Observe the Breath

Choose a comfortable position and begin to observe your natural inhale, exhale and pauses in between. Breathing through the nostrils, notice

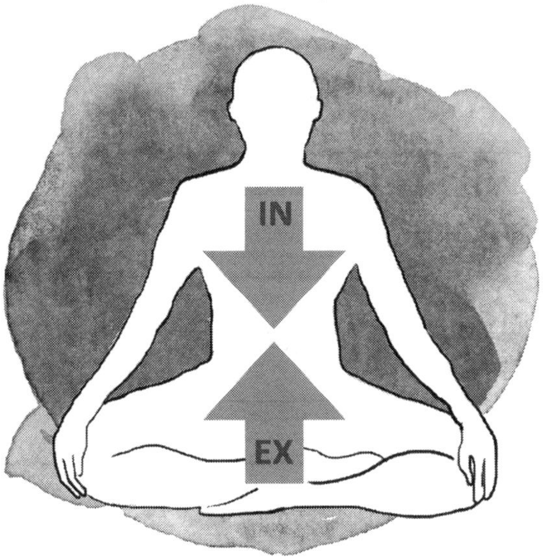

how your body moves as you breathe in and out. As you inhale, observe how the air moves from the nose through the throat and down into your lungs. As you exhale, notice how the breath moves up from your lungs, through the throat and out your nose.

Practice 2: Begin *Ujjāyī* Breathing

Breathe through the nostrils with a slight constriction in the back of the throat. This technique will produce an audible, whispering sound. For more detailed instructions on *ujjāyī*, refer back to chapter 13 on Breath and Movement. Begin the exhale with a firm but gentle contraction of the abdomen, drawing the navel toward the spine. On inhale, expand your chest slightly and extend the spine. When done properly, *ujjāyī* slows down the breath, creates a longer inhale and exhale and helps direct the breath to the lower third of the lungs.

In the following ratio-*pranayama* practices, be sure to maintain a comfortable *ujjāyī* throughout.

Practice 3: Equalizing the Inhale and Exhale

As you continue with *ujjāyī* breathing, begin to count the length of your exhale. Next, count the length of your inhale. If one part of the breath is longer than the other, shorten it, making the ratio between inhale and exhale equal. Finally, add a short pause after both inhale and exhale and continue for 6 more breaths.

Practice 4: Extending the Exhale

Here, our goal is to extend the exhale to twice as long as the inhale. Begin with an inhale and exhale that are equal in length and comfortable. Although in the practice below we have chosen to begin with a three second inhale and exhale, the actual starting length may be shorter or longer, depending on what's comfortable for you.

In this practice, the beginning ratio between the length of the inhale and exhale is equal (line #1). Remember, always include a natural pause of 1 or 2 seconds between the inhale and exhale. Each round increases the exhale by one second until we reach our goal (line #4).

Round	Ratio in Seconds IN.HOLD.EX.HOLD	Number of Breaths
# 1	3.0.3.0	2
# 2	3.0.4.0	2
# 3	3.0.5.0	2
# 4	3.0.6.0	6 (goal ratio)

Practice 5: Extending the Inhale

Having extended your exhale, you can now extend your inhale using the same process. Begin with the length of the exhale you achieved in the previous practice.

Round	Ratio in Seconds IN.HOLD.EX.HOLD	Number of Breaths
# 1	3.0.6.0	2
# 2	4.0.6.0	2
# 3	5.0.6.0	2
# 4	6.0.6.0	6 (goal ratio)

Practice 6: Introducing Hold after Exhale

Now that you have extended both parts of the breath, you are ready to practice holding after exhale. Each time you suspend the breath, remember to observe and release any tension you may be experiencing.

Round	Ratio in Seconds IN.HOLD.EX.HOLD	Number of Breaths
# 1	4.0.4.2	2
# 2	4.0.4.3	2
# 3	4.0.4.4	6 (goal ratio)
# 4	4.0.4.0	2

Practice 7: Introducing Holds after Inhale

Once you are comfortable with the hold after the exhale, you are ready to extend the hold after the inhale.

Round	Ratio in Seconds IN.HOLD.EX.HOLD	Number of Breaths
# 1	4.2.4.0	2
# 2	4.3.4.0	2
# 3	4.4.4.0	6 (goal ratio)
# 4	4.0.4.0	2

**Practice 8:
Using Holds after Inhale and Exhale**

Now that you have experience with all four parts of the breath, you are ready to challenge yourself with the following practice.

Round	Ratio in Seconds IN.HOLD.EX.HOLD	Number of Breaths
# 1	4.0.4.0	2
# 2	4.2.4.2	2
# 3	4.3.4.3	2
# 4	4.4.4.4	6 (goal ratio)

Practice 9: Extending the Exhale by Using Holds

Once holds have become comfortable, they can be used as a mechanism to lengthen the breath. Let's start with the hold after the exhale. On round #2, add a hold after exhale of 3 seconds. On round #3, add that to the length of the exhale increasing it by 3 seconds.

Round	Ratio in Seconds IN.HOLD.EX.HOLD	Number of Breaths
# 1	5.0.5.0	3
# 2	5.0.5.3	3
# 3	5.0.8.0	6 (goal ratio)

Practice 10: Extending the Inhale by Using Holds

The same principle can be applied to extending the inhale with holds.

Round	Ratio in Seconds IN.HOLD.EX.HOLD	Number of Breaths
# 1	5.0.8.0	3
# 2	5.3.8.0	3
# 3	8.0.8.0	6 (goal ratio)

Energetics of Ratio

The above practices are examples of how to use ratio in *prāṇāyāma*. As you may have experienced, the practice using equal inhale and exhale created a balanced, *samana* feeling. The ratios which lengthened the exhale and hold after exhale resulted in a more relaxed, *laṅghana* feeling. This type of practice can be used to help us unwind after a hard day's work or lead to a better night's sleep. The practices which lengthened the inhale and the hold after inhale, promoted a more energetic *bṛṁhaṇa* feeling. This type of practice helps to reduce feelings of fatigue or lethargy.

Try each practice for a week and take note of its effects. Has your breath become smoother and longer? Do you have more energy? Is your mind a little clearer? Are you sleeping better?

Introduction to *Prāṇāyāma* Techniques

As stated earlier, in *prāṇāyāma,* we can consciously constrict or valve the breath through the throat, tongue or nostrils. When done properly, these valving techniques along with *mudrās,* make our normal breath longer and smoother. They can be used independently or in different combinations. First, we will highlight techniques using the tongue and throat to regulate the flow of breath.

There are 2 techniques using the tongue as a valve, one is *śītalī* and the other is *śītkārī*. In *śītalī prāṇāyāma,* we control the breath by curling the tongue like a straw and inhaling through it. If curling the tongue is not possible (some people are genetically unable to do so), try inhaling with the tip of the tongue pressed against the back of the teeth. This technique is called *śītkārī* and, like *śītalī,* it has a cooling effect on the body and mind. The process is as follows.

Tongue Breathing Techniques

Śītalī

In this technique we inhale through the curled tongue and exhale *ujjāyī*.

- Sit with a straight spine. Start by tucking the chin slightly toward the chest.
- Curl the tongue and extend it like a straw.
- Inhale through the curled tongue while slowly raising the chin as far as comfortable.
- At the end of the inhale, pause, close the mouth and relax the tongue.
- With the mouth closed, exhale *ujjāyī* while lowering the chin back to the tucked position.

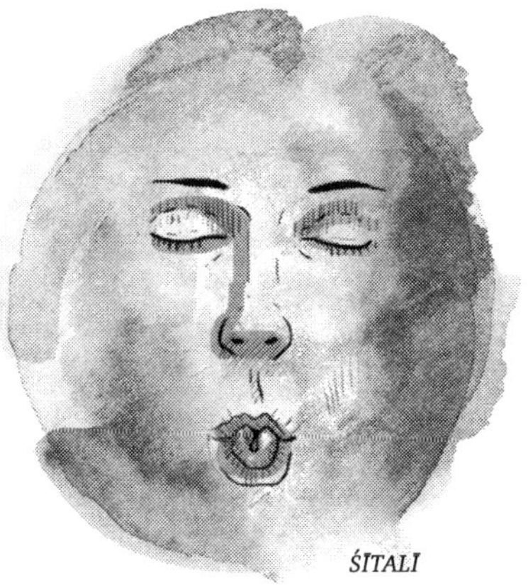

ŚĪTALĪ

Breathing through the curled tongue provides a cooling effect for our bodies, minds and emotions.

Śītkārī

- In this technique we exhale *ujjāyī* and touch the tongue to the back of the teeth on inhale.
- Sit with a straight spine. Start by tucking the chin slightly toward the chest.
- With a slightly open mouth, press the tip of the tongue against the back of the upper front teeth and inhale, making a hissing sound while simultaneously lifting the chin as far as comfortable.

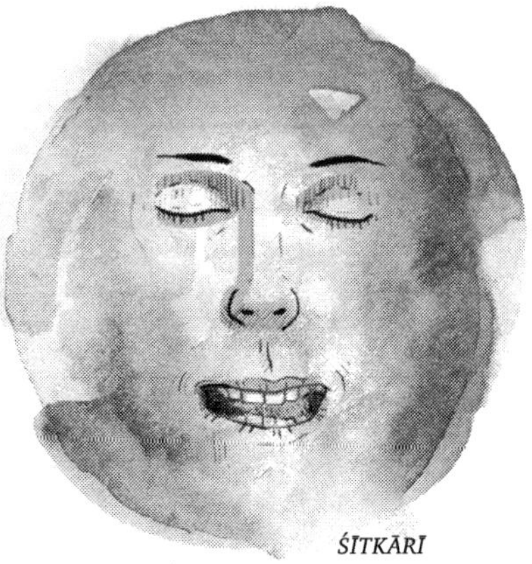

ŚĪTKĀRĪ

- At the end of the inhale, pause, relax the tongue, close the mouth and exhale *ujjāyī* while lowering the chin back to the tucked position.

Śītkārī provides the same cooling effect as *śītalī*.

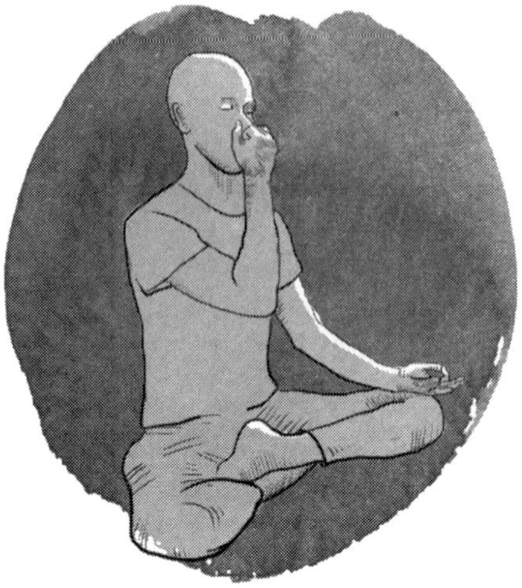

Nostril Breathing Techniques

Next, we will discuss nostril techniques and how to valve the breath using *mudrās*. These techniques are incredibly powerful, as they stimulate the oldest part of the brain, the olfactory lobe. This area is linked to our most basic survival skills, such as, avoiding danger, hunting for food and choosing sexual partners. Many believe that breathing through alternating nostrils integrates our analytical and creative abilities by balancing the right and left hemispheres of the brain.

All nostril breathing involves inhaling or exhaling while partially closing one nostril and completely blocking the other with *mṛgi mudrā*. Refer to the picture below or the above directions for this *mudrā*.

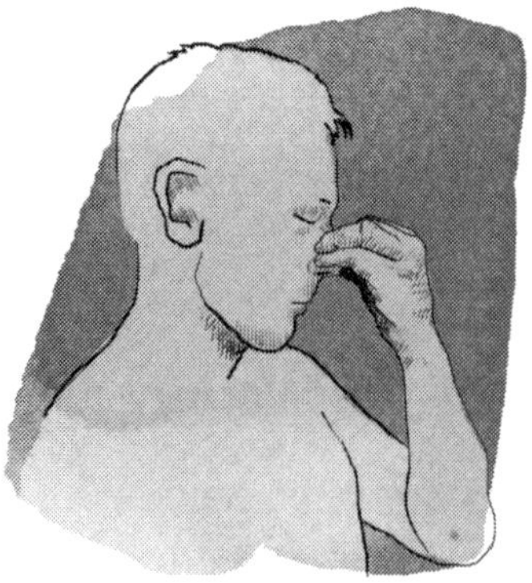

Although there are other nostril techniques, we will cover *anuloma ujjāyī, viloma ujjāyī and nāḍī śodhana*. These techniques can either have a balancing or heating effect.

Anuloma Ujjāyī

In this technique we breathe using *ujjāyī* on the inhale and through alternating nostrils on exhale:

- Sit with a straight spine, left hand in *cin mudrā*, right hand in *mṛgi mudrā*.
- Inhale *ujjāyī*, pause.
- During the pause, raise your right hand and place your thumb on the lower part of the right nostril, completely blocking off the air flow. Rest the last two fingers on the cartilage of the left nostril, creating a partial opening.
- Slowly exhale through the partial opening of the left nostril while keeping the right nostril completely blocked.
- Bring the hand back to your lap during the pause after exhale.
- Inhale *ujjāyī*, pause.
- During the pause, raise your hand and place your ring and pinkie finger on the lower part of the left nostril, completely blocking off the air flow. Rest your thumb on the cartilage of your right nostril, creating a partial opening.
- Slowly exhale through the partial opening of the right nostril while keeping the left nostril completely blocked.
- Bring the hand back to your lap during the pause after exhale. This completes one cycle or round of *anuloma ujjāyī prāṇāyāma*.

Simplified instructions for anuloma ujjāyī:
inhale *ujjāyī*, exhale left nostril,
inhale *ujjāyī*, exhale right nostril.

Viloma Ujjāyī

This technique uses *ujjāyī* breathing only on the exhale and the alternate nostril on the inhale — the opposite of *anuloma ujjāyī*.

- Sit with a straight spine, left hand in *cin mudrā*, right hand in *mṛgi mudrā*.
- Exhale *ujjāyī*, pause.
- During the pause, raise your right hand and place your thumb on the lower part of the right nostril, completely blocking off the air flow. Rest your ring and pinky fingers on the cartilage of your left nostril, creating a partial opening.
- Slowly inhale through the partial opening of the left nostril while keeping the right nostril completely blocked.
- Bring the right hand back to your lap during the pause after inhale.
- Exhale *ujjāyī*, pause.
- During the pause, raise your right hand and completely block your left nostril with the pinky and ring fingers, inhale through the partial opening created by the thumb resting on the cartilage of your right nostril.
- Bring the hand back to your lap during the pause after inhale.
- Exhale *ujjāyī*, pause. This completes one cycle or round of *viloma ujjāyī prāṇāyāma*.

> ***Simplified instructions for viloma ujjāyī:***
> inhale left nostril, exhale *ujjāyī*,
> inhale right nostril, exhale *ujjāyī*.

Nāḍī Śodhana

Once you are comfortable with *anuloma* and *viloma ujjāyī*, you are ready for *nāḍī śodhana*, a technique that uses alternate nostril breathing on both inhale and exhale.

- Sit with a straight spine, left hand in *cin mudrā* and the right hand in *mṛgi mudrā*.
- Maintaining *mṛgi mudrā*, bring the right hand to the nose, where it will remain throughout the practice.
- Inhale through the partially opened left nostril while keeping your right nostril completely blocked.
- Exhale through the partially opened right nostril while keeping your left nostril completely blocked.
- Inhale through the partially opened right nostril while keeping your left nostril completely blocked.
- Exhale through the partially opened left nostril while keeping your right nostril completely blocked. This completes one round of *nāḍī śodhana prāṇāyāma*.

> ***Simplified instructions for nāḍī śodhana:***
> inhale left nostril, exhale right nostril,
> inhale right nostril, exhale left nostril.

On a cautionary note, be gentle with yourself when doing *prāṇāyāma*. Forcing these techniques could result in shortness of breath and mental agitation, thus defeating the aim of practice. Because each technique has its own purpose and energetic effect, a teacher is invaluable in helping to determine what is most useful for you and how to achieve it.

Once you are familiar with these techniques, the chart on next the page serves as a quick reference guide, along with the contraindications for these practices.

Mouth Breathing	*Throat Breathing*	*Nostril Breathing*	*Nostril/Throat Combination*
śītalī inhale through curled tongue (exhale *ujjāyī*) ***śītkārī*** inhale through tongue pressed against back of teeth (exhale *ujjāyī*)	***ujjāyī*** throat breathing	***nāḍī śodhana*** alternate nostril breathing: inhale left nostril, exhale right nostril, inhale right nostril, exhale left nostril	***anuloma ujjāyī*** inhale *ujjāyī*, exhale alternate nostrils ***viloma ujjāyī*** inhale alternate nostrils, exhale *ujjāyī*
Avoid if you have dry mouth.	Avoid if you have a sore throat.	Avoid if you have a cold or congestion.	Avoid if you have a sore throat, cold or congestion.

Tools to Enhance your *Prāṇāyāma* Practices

In *prāṇāyāma*, the focus is always on the breath. Following are two tools that can be used to complement your practice, *bhāvana* and *mantra*.

Bhāvana is a technique in which we visualize specific images or concepts to help clarify and move us closer to our goals. Following is an example of how to use this tool to create more energy and vitality:

- As you inhale, visualize the energy of the sun being drawn into the body.
- On the hold after inhale, allow it to expand and nourish the system.
- On exhale, visualize letting go of any obstacles to that vitality.

Mantra is the silent recitation of meaningful phrases used to intensify the effect of a *prāṇāyāma* practice. For example instead of counting the length of the breath you can use *mantra*.

- Mentally recite as you inhale, "Let the sun nourish me."
- On hold after inhale, recite "Let the sun nourish me."
- On exhale, recite "Let the sun nourish me."

The detailed instructions contained in this chapter are meant to serve merely as an introduction to *prāṇāyāma*. Our hope is that you will cultivate a regular practice and experience the beauty and power of this highly transformational *yogic* tool for yourself. Further instruction on refinement and individual application of *prāṇāyāma* requires the guidance of a qualified teacher.

To Sum Up:

- Shallow, irregular breathing can negatively impact our nervous system, overall health and mental stability.
- Slow, deep, conscious breathing helps cultivate the stable mind and balanced emotions necessary for meditation.
- All *prāṇāyāma* practices consist of regulating the breath to make it longer and smoother than normal, unconscious breathing.
- There are four parts of the breath: inhale, hold, exhale, hold.
- Ratio is the length of all four parts of the breath and their relationship to each another.
- There are three physical locations to valve the breath: throat, tongue and nostrils.
- Working with any part of the breath should never distort any other part of the breath.
- *Mudrās* are hand positions with symbolic and/or practical applications.
- We have discussed six techniques for *prāṇāyāma*. They are:
    1. *ujjāyī*
    2. *śītalī*
    3. *śītkārī*
    4. *anuloma ujjāyī*
    5. *viloma ujjāyī*
    6. *nāḍī śodhana*
- *Bhāvana* and *mantra* can be used to enhance *prāṇāyāma* practice.

CHAPTER 19

Cultivating a Stable Mind: Meditation/Fifth, Sixth, Seventh & Eighth Limbs

Today, *āsana* is taught everywhere from fitness centers to colleges, prisons, hospitals and an ever-growing number of *Yoga* studios. Many practitioners who have only been exposed to *āsana* equate *Yoga* with performing postures. Classically, however, the primary intention of the physical practice was to enable the practitioner to sit comfortably, focus the mind and, ultimately, to meditate.

In the *Yoga Sūtra*, meditation is described as the ability to consciously choose an appropriate object and sustain attention on that object for an extended period of time. This object serves as a focal point for the mind. It can be external, such as a picture of someone we admire, or internal, like the calming flow of our breath. With consistent practice, meditation enables us to control the mind which improves our attitude and leads to positive, life-changing results.

In this chapter, we will cover the reasons to meditate, the five states of mind described by the sage, Vyasa, in his commentary on the *Yoga Sūtras*, and how those states of mind relate to meditation. We will also discuss the stages and tools of meditation, as well as the value of creating ritual in our practice.

Purposes to Meditate

Regular meditation has been shown to promote a variety of health benefits, including reduced stress, better sleep, improved pain management and stronger immune functions. Though all the health benefits provide ample incentive, there are more deep-rooted reasons to practice meditation.

In fact, the underlying aim of all *Yoga* practice was to understand and, ultimately, experience the true nature, structure and potential of the human mind. To this end, meditation was the primary tool. The lineage of T. Krishnamacharya, in which this book is based, draws from the ancient texts to present five fundamental purposes to practice meditation: power, knowledge, healing, personal responsibilities (*dharma*) and spirituality. For meditation to be truly effective, we must first be clear on which of these five is the purpose of our practice.

Power

Power enables us to accomplish something that was not formerly possible. This includes anything from attaining new physical abilities to achieving mastery in a particular area of our lives. For example, if we wish to become a better athlete we can meditate on the skills and strategies of the sport in which we are interested or visualize ourselves excelling in that activity. We could also choose to focus on the energy, perseverance or dedication of a sports figure we admire. In order to cultivate strength of character, we could meditate on a person who lives their life with truthfulness and integrity.

Knowledge

A second purpose for meditating is to gain knowledge, to learn more about something that piques our interest. This could be self-knowledge or more information about something outside ourselves. To gain knowledge about something outside ourselves, such as learning a foreign language, we might choose to meditate on its vocabulary, grammar and rhythm. This can be done by having a teacher guide us, reading books or watching movies in which the language is spoken. A dedicated gardener might choose to spend many hours throughout the year meditating on the seasonal changes to understand what is required for the flowers or vegetables to grow. On a more subtle level, they could gain insight on how to flourish in their own life.

Healing

Another purpose for meditation is healing. Meditation can be used to reduce the symptoms of suffering, address their causes and, ultimately, change our relationship with an ailment or disease. By spending time in nature, meditating on the sun and the nourishing qualities of fresh air, we could achieve a myriad of health benefits and greater sense of well-being. Healing might also occur by meditating on our positive relationships and their ability to support us, warm our hearts and soothe our souls.

Personal Responsibilities *(dharma)*

Still another reason to meditate is to understand our personal responsibilities or *dharma*. Due to the complexity of our lives, we are often unclear about which responsibilities are truly our own, as well as which ones should be a priority at any given time. The primary goals of *dharma* meditation are to gain clarity on what, exactly, our responsibilities are and to maintain the single-minded focus needed to fulfill them. The more our actions are aligned with our *dharma*, the more we experience a deeper sense of joy and accomplishment.

According to *Yoga*, the first *dharma* is practicing appropriate self-care to ensure that we are healthy and able to carry out our responsibilities to others and to the environment. A mother's primary *dharmic* meditation is to focus on providing proper care for her young children over any other responsibilities. As the children mature, the mother's *dharmic* meditation will change to help them navigate through their lives.

The *dharma* of a son or daughter could be to meditate on the needs of their aging parents. A teacher's meditation might be focusing on the strengths and weaknesses of their students in order to provide appropriate guidance. A citizen's *dharmic* meditation might be to identify their role in maintaining a healthy ecology.

Spirituality

The final purpose of meditation is spirituality. For some, this means participation in an organized religion and devotion to a specific deity or deities. For others, spirituality is a connection with something greater, wiser and more powerful than themselves, such as nature or the soul within. However we view spirituality, meditation will deepen and enhance our experience of it. For example, if we are religious, meditation might entail praying to a chosen deity for the improved health of a loved one. Meditating on the breath can create an awareness of, or deepen our connection to, the spirit within.

We have presented the five purposes for meditation from our tradition as though they are distinct from each another. In our everyday lives, they often combine and overlap. If you are unclear about what the purpose of your meditation should be, once again, the help of a teacher is invaluable.

The Five States of Mind

Today, there is an endless barrage of stimuli competing for our attention. This, combined with our own tendencies towards distraction, explains why many find it daunting to even approach the practice of meditation. T. Krishnamacharya addressed the challenges to meditation by describing the five possible states of mind:

At times, our minds are completely **agitated and distracted**. When we become overwhelmed by events, real or imagined, in our daily lives, we find it impossible to focus.

Alternatively, the mind can become **dull or depleted**. In this state, we experience doubt, hopelessness or a lack of motivation. We find ourselves unable to generate the energy needed to solve problems and be productive.

A far more common state is when the mind **vacillates between attention and distraction**. Here, we do have the ability to focus our attention, but only intermittently.

In the fourth state of mind, although there is still a degree of distraction, we are able to **consciously direct attention** on a chosen object for an extended period of time.

Finally, there is a rare, elevated state in which we are no longer affected by external or internal distractions. Here, the mind is **wholly absorbed** in the object of focus.

Knowledge of the five states of mind gives us a deeper understanding of our habitual mental patterns as well our true potential. With increased awareness and sustained practice, we can develop the degree of control needed to begin the meditation process.

Stages of Meditation

A recurring theme in the *Yoga Sūtras* is the progression from gross to subtle. In the Eight Limbs Model, Patañjali prescribes the consistent practice of *āsana* and *prāṇāyāma*, the outer limbs, as a preparation for the inner, more subtle practices, *pratyāhāra, dhāraṇā, dhyāna* and *samādhi*.

A prerequisite for meditation is *pratyāhāra*, the ability to control the senses and choose an object on which to focus (*dhāraṇā*). Over time, sustaining this focus deepens our connection with the object (*dhyāna*). Eventually, we experience *samādhi*, a state of complete absorption with the object. Let's take a more in-depth look at these steps.

Pratyāhāra

Our senses are essential for both our survival and enjoyment of life. They link our internal and external worlds. Depending on how they are used, the senses can either help us achieve our goals or highjack our best intentions.

Pratyāhāra, Aṣṭāṅga Yoga's fifth limb, is the ability to appreciate the senses, while relegating them to their proper place, as instruments of our deeper consciousness rather than as a distracting force. As a result we are able to direct our attention with greater ease.

Pratyāhāra may be achieved through the deliberate practice of sensory control or it may happen as a result of practicing *Yoga*'s first four limbs: *yama, niyama, āsana and prāṇāyāma*. However it occurs, control of our senses is a prerequisite for choosing an object of focus for meditation.

Robert's Story:

One morning when I was first learning to meditate, the intoxicating aroma of almond biscotti nearly distracted me from my practice. For a moment, I considered following the smell to its source. Remembering what I had been taught, I made a conscious choice to practice *pratyāhāra* and continue with my meditation. I was able to reap the benefits of this decision all day long.

Often, our minds are unconsciously driven by what we see, hear, feel, taste and smell. We find ourselves endlessly surfing the internet, texting while driving or mindlessly eating an entire bag of potato chips. Only when we are able to control the senses, can we begin the process of meditation.

Dhāraṇā

The first step in *Yoga* meditation is *dhāraṇā*, choosing an object of focus. The *sūtras* teach that we absorb the qualities of whatever we give our attention to. Therefore, what we choose to focus on is of utmost importance. Also, what we link with serves as a symbol of what we wish to achieve or cultivate in our lives. We can meditate on something external, like the sun or a picture of someone we admire. Or we can meditate on something internal, such as compassion, gratitude or a higher power.

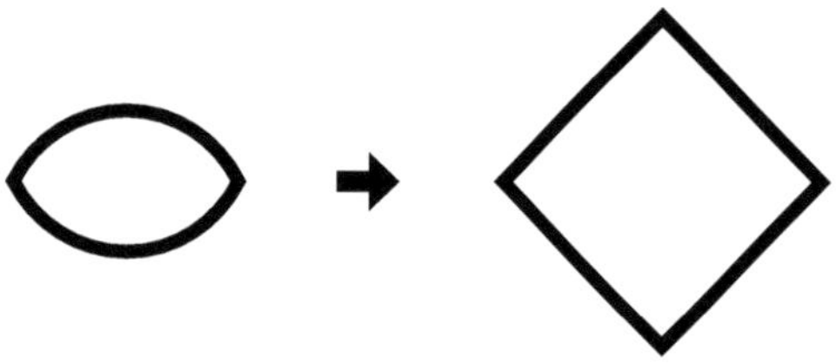

Mind Senses Object

Dhyāna

Having chosen the object of focus, the next step is *dhyāna*, the heart of meditation. It is through this sustained focus that we develop a deep connection leading to a powerful relationship with the object. As a result, we gain more knowledge of the object itself, greater understanding of our own minds and, with consistent practice, insights into that which is beyond the mind.

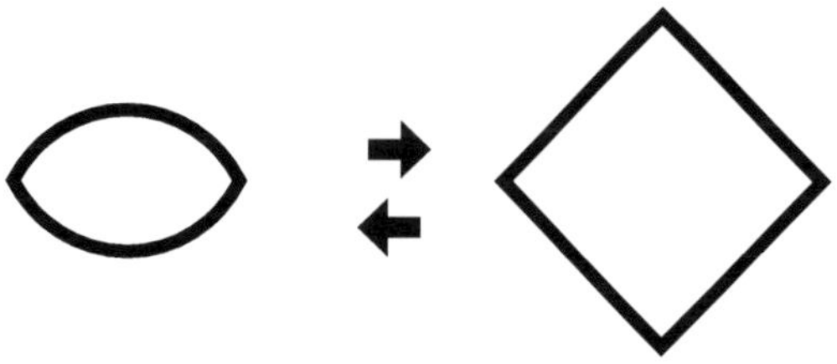

Mind Object

For example, if we choose to meditate on the sun, we link with the sun's power to illuminate and nourish all living things. This meditation also offers insight into the healing energy of nature and how we can best use it to improve our lives.

As we attempt to create this relationship with the chosen object, many of us find it difficult to sustain our attention. This may be because the mind is not adequately prepared for meditation and we need to practice a bit more *āsana* or *prāṇāyāma*. Another possibility is that we need to reflect and reevaluate the object we have chosen. Whatever the reason, struggling to meditate can actually increase mental agitation. Therefore, once again, guidance from a qualified teacher is invaluable.

Samādhi

Once we have chosen an appropriate object of meditation and successfully sustained a link with it, we may reach *samādhi*, the state of complete absorption with the object. In this final stage of meditation, we experience a heightened state of awareness in which there is an altered sense of time and feelings of self-consciousness are diminished. As this is a progressive process which develops over time, we must continue to deepen our connection with the object of focus in order for *samādhi* to occur.

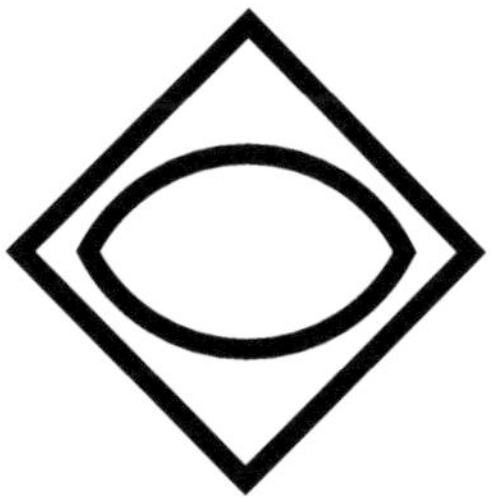

Mind/Object Merged

For instance, if we were to reach the state of *samādhi* in the sun meditation, we would feel as though we had completely absorbed the sun's nourishing power. As a result, we might experience a newfound vigor for life or realize our potential for increased health and well-being.

Here's a simple example to help understand the three stages of meditation. Let's say you want to learn how to play a musical instrument. The very first step is deciding which one you'd like to play. Choosing the guitar over all the other possible instruments is *dhāraṇā*. Over time, with consistent practice, you develop a relationship with the instrument. As a result of this connection, you would not only discover the range of the guitar's capabilities, but also become aware of, and deepen, your love for the instrument as well. This is *dhyāna*. Eventually, this connection goes so deep, it is as though you no longer feel any separation between yourself, the guitar and the music. This is the state of total absorption, *samādhi*. To get a true sense of this state you need only watch a master musician perform when they are "in the zone."

Whatever object we choose, the ultimate aim of *Yoga* meditation is to create a state of mind in which we experience and are guided by our deepest intelligence on a daily basis. Many names have been given to this "inner GPS": including *puruṣa*, consciousness, the perceiver, spirit and the soul. Though much has been written in an attempt to describe this state, it is ultimately something that each individual can only experience for themselves. To quote T.K.V. Desikachar, "If a man is lost in the woods, it is of no value to describe the banquet waiting for him at his home. Our job is to give him a map so he can find his way there." Meditation is that map.

Fundamental Tools of Meditation

Bhāvana

Imagination is an innate human ability. If you ask a child about their future, they will describe in vivid detail what they want to become, such as a firefighter, superhero or an astronaut, etc. *Bhāvana* is a powerful *yogic* tool in which we use our imagination to clarify our values and visualize an object for our meditation. With *bhāvana*, we imagine what it will look and feel like after we have already created what we want.

We can observe that everything in the material world, other than nature, started out as a visualization or *bhāvana* in someone's mind. The discovery of electricity, the invention of the computer, and the ability to put an astronaut on the moon are examples of the power of *bhāvana*. This power is greatly magnified when the *bhāvana* is: positive, concrete, and specific. Let's explore these three qualities.

- **Positive** — It is far more effective to focus on creating or increasing what we do want, rather than eliminating or reducing what we don't. It is more useful to visualize ourselves increasing our vitality and enthusiasm rather than reducing our disease and depression. Patañjali defines this as cultivating an opposite perspective.
- **Concrete** — What many find challenging is translating abstract concepts into observable behaviors. For instance, we might decide that our goal is to become more compassionate, but we have trouble visualizing exactly what that would look like. An example of how to make this concept more concrete would be to visualize ourselves engaged in an actual compassionate act, such as helping a friend in need or doing volunteer work.
- **Specific** — Finally, the more precise and vivid our visualizations, the more they evoke the emotions that will, ultimately, fuel our actions. Visualizing ourselves working at a nearby food bank three days a month, seeing the faces of people we are feeding turn from sad and hungry to happy and fed, will evoke in us feelings of compassion.

To reiterate, when our *bhāvana* is positive, concrete and specific, it has the potential to create dramatic changes in our lives.

Mudrā

As you may recall from the chapter on *prāṇāyāma, mudrās* are hand positions in which we arrange the fingers in a specific way or place the hands on a specific part of the body to create a closed circuit of energy. In meditation, *mudrās* are also used to provide a tangible point of focus for our minds. In the next chapter we will use *cin mudrā* and two additional *mudrās* to achieve these effects. They are:

Saṅkalpa Mudrā

In *saṅkalpa mudrā*, we clasp the hands together and place them on the right knee, left hand on the bottom, right on top. This *mudrā* is a symbol of our commitment to follow through with our practice. It is combined with a spoken statement of our intention, and is often used as the starting point for a meditation practice.

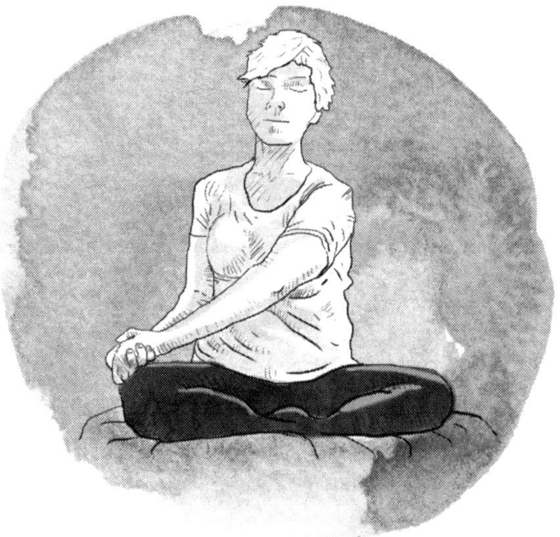

SAṄKALPA MUDRĀ

Dhyāna Mudrā

In *dhyāna mudrā*, we bring both hands to our lap, placing the left hand on the bottom and our right hand on top, palms facing up. This *mudrā* symbolizes our receptivity to the teachings, the teacher and all that our meditation has to offer.

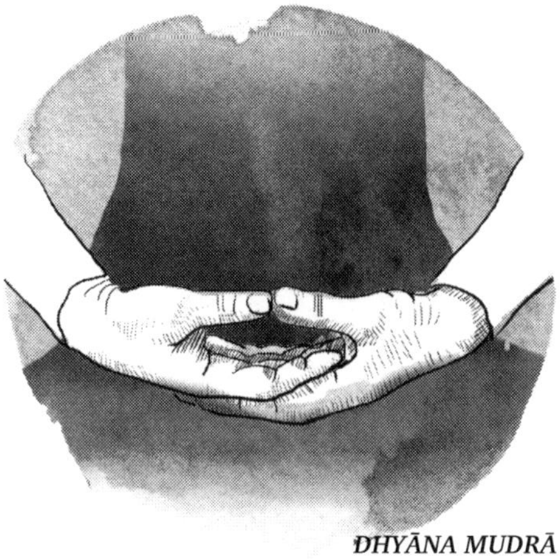

DHYĀNA MUDRĀ

Ritual

Many individuals have experienced difficulty cultivating a consistent meditation practice. We have found that creating meaningful rituals to begin our practice makes it easier.

A ritual is a sequence of actions performed in a particular order to signal the end of one activity and the beginning of another. When the same ritual is performed regularly, it makes everyday events more meaningful. Examples of how rituals already enhance our lives might include enjoying a bath at the end of a workday, having a cake to celebrate a birthday or connecting with a friend over a weekly cup of coffee.

There are many ways to create meaningful meditation rituals. For example:

- Set aside a certain time each day to turn off the phone and computer to minimize distractions.
- Prepare a dedicated space with your mat and cushion.
- Set an altar with your object of focus, candles or flowers, to create a peaceful ambience.
- Perform a short *āsana* and *prāṇāyāma* practice to prepare yourself for meditation.

The practice of meditation is a journey that enriches our lives and gives us more purpose and direction. It makes the mind increasingly focused and inwardly directed. When we develop a consistent meditation practice, we find it easier to observe the nature of our hearts and minds. Over time, meditation informs our behavior and deepens our connection with our own spirit and the world around us.

In the next chapter, we will explore the various tools of meditation, describe their appropriate applications and give step-by-step instructions for designing specific meditation practices.

To Sum Up:

- Classically, there are five purposes for meditation:
  1. power
  2. knowledge
  3. healing
  4. personal responsibilities/*dharma*
  5. spirituality
- There are five distinct states of minds on the path to meditation:
  1. agitated and distracted
  2. dull
  3. vacillating between attention and distraction
  4. concentration
  5. total absorption
- The *Yoga Sūtras* state *āsana* and *prāṇāyāma* are prerequisites to prepare the mind for meditation.
- There are four Stages of Meditation:
  1. *pratyāhāra* (controlling the senses)
  2. *dhāraṇā* (the ability to choose an appropriate object)
  3. *dhyāna* (the ability to sustain focus on and develop a relationship with the object over time)
  4. *samādhi* (complete absorption in the object of focus)
- Fundamental tools of meditation:
  1. *Bhāvana*/visualization is a powerful tool for choosing an object of focus.
  2. Rituals make ordinary events meaningful and our meditation practice easier.
  3. *Mudrās* can provide a tangible point of focus for our minds.

CHAPTER 20

Developing a Meditation Practice

In the previous chapter, we presented the stages of meditation, its purposes as well as the fundamental tools needed to support a meditation practice.

In order for a meditation practice to be effective, it must be repeated over an extended period of time. Though some positive effects will be felt immediately, it is only when we cultivate a consistent, long-term relationship with our practice that we will experience its deep, transformational benefits in our daily lives.

We have designed four short practices for you to experience both the process and effects of meditation. As each one has a specific intention, we have chosen the ratio *prāṇāyāma* that matches the purpose of the practice. Remember to begin by preparing a space where you will not be distracted.

Meditation Practices
Practice 1

The intention of this practice is **power**, specifically the power of increased confidence.

- **Step one**: *dhāraṇā* — choosing an object of focus.

Choose a person in your life or an historical figure who, you feel embodies strength and confidence. Place an image, picture or statue of this person directly in front of you, at eye level.

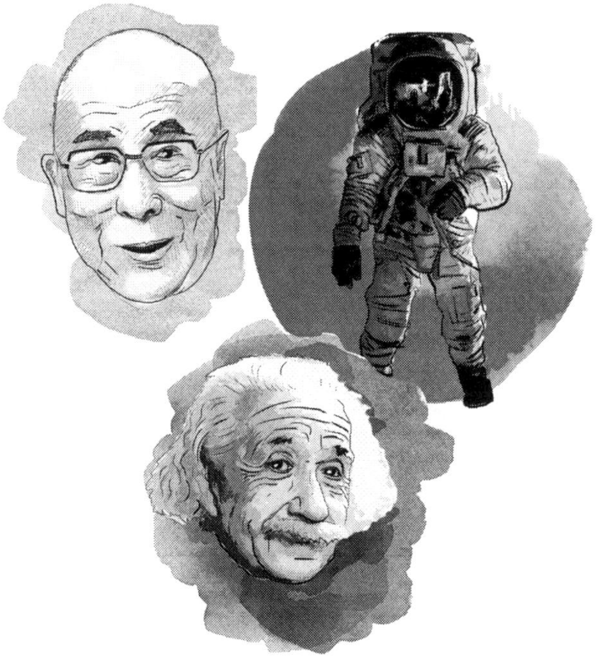

- **Step two**: *āsana* — prepare the body.

Do a short practice emphasizing backbends to create a *bṛṁhaṇa* effect.

- Step three: *prāṇāyāma* — prepare the breath.

Sit either on the floor or in a chair. Begin with some comfortable, *ujjāyī* breaths, making the inhale and exhale the same length. Increase the hold after inhale 1 second every 3 breaths until the hold is the same length as the inhale.

Round	Ratio in Seconds IN.HOLD.EX.HOLD	Number of Breaths
# 1	4.0.4.0	3
# 2	4.2.4.0	3
# 3	4.3.4.0	3
# 4	4.4.4.0	3 (goal ratio)

- **Step four:** state your *saṅkalpa* — intention.

While gazing at the image, place your hands in *saṅkalpa mudrā* and repeat your intention aloud: "I commit to completing this practice; may it empower me and fill me with confidence."

- **Step five:** *dhyāna* — meditation.

Place your hands in *cin mudrā*. Gaze at the picture until you have created a link. Then, close your eyes and hold the image of the person in your mind. Feel yourself taking in the qualities of confidence and strength. Continue to deepen your connection with these qualities and observe them in yourself.

- **Step six:** *samādhi* — absorption.

Having absorbed the qualities of strength and confidence, sit and savor the experience. This could be several minutes or longer. Remember, achieving a state of *samādhi* takes time and requires regular practice.

- **Step seven:** delinking.

When you are ready to delink from the object of meditation, take six *ujjāyī* breaths, making your exhale twice as long as your inhale.

Round	Ratio in Seconds IN.HOLD.EX.HOLD	Number of Breaths
# 1	4.0.8.0	6

- **Step eight**: transition.

Maintain this focused state of mind as you perform some gentle *āsana* to reconnect with your body. Express gratitude for what you have received from the practice and set your intention to bring those feelings and qualities into your daily life.

Practice 2

The intention of this practice is **healing**, specifically, to reduce the effects of stress.

- **Step one:** *dhāraṇā* — choosing an object of focus.

Choose a picture of something from the natural world that, for you, suggests the qualities of calmness and beauty — for example, a still, blue lake. Place the image in front of you at eye level.

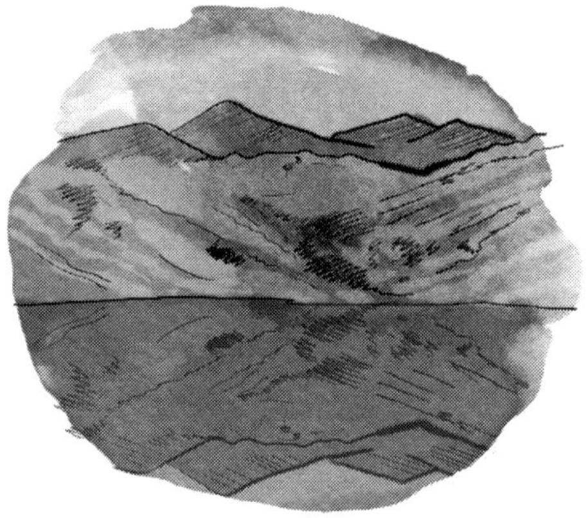

- **Step two:** *āsana* — prepare the body.

Do a short practice emphasizing gentle forward bends and twists that lengthen the exhale to create a *laṅghana* effect.

- **Step three:** *prāṇāyāma* — prepare the breath.

Take a comfortable, seated position, either on the floor or in a chair. Begin with some comfortable, *ujjāyī* breaths, making the inhale and exhale the same length. After a few breaths, start increasing the exhale by 2 counts every 4 breaths, until it is twice the length of the inhale.

Round	Ratio in Seconds IN.HOLD.EX.HOLD	Number of Breaths
# 1	4.0.4.0	4
# 2	4.0.6.0	4
# 3	4.0.8.0	4

- **Step four:** *saṅkalpa* — state your intention.

While gazing at the image, place your hands in *saṅkalpa mudrā* and repeat your intention aloud; "I commit to completing this practice, may it calm me and bring me to a state of deep relaxation."

- **Step five:** *dhyāna* — meditation.

Place your hands in *dhyāna mudrā* and gaze at the picture until you feel you have created a link with this beautiful, natural scene. Then close your eyes, hold the image in your mind and begin to absorb the qualities of stillness and peace. Continue to deepen your connection with these qualities until you observe them in yourself.

- **Step six:** *samādhi* — absorption.

When you feel you have fully absorbed the quality of relaxation, sit and savor the experience. Once again, remember, meditation is a progressive process which will develop over time.

- **Step seven:** delinking.

When you feel you are ready to delink from the object of meditation, take six *ujjāyī* breaths with your exhale twice as long as your inhale.

Round	Ratio in Seconds IN.HOLD.EX.HOLD	Number of Breaths
# 1	4.0.8.0	6

- **Step eight:** transition.

Maintain this focused state of mind as you perform some gentle *āsana* to reconnect with your body. Set your intention to bring the qualities you have absorbed into your daily life.

Practice 3

The intention of this practice is ***dharma***, to clarify the actions needed to fulfill a specific responsibility in our lives. In this practice, we have chosen the sun, representing clarity, as our object of meditation. This clarity will guide us in taking the steps needed to realize our *dharma*.

- **Step one:** *dhāraṇā* — choosing an object of focus.

Find a representation of the sun (a picture or an object) to symbolize this clarity. Place it in front of you at eye level.

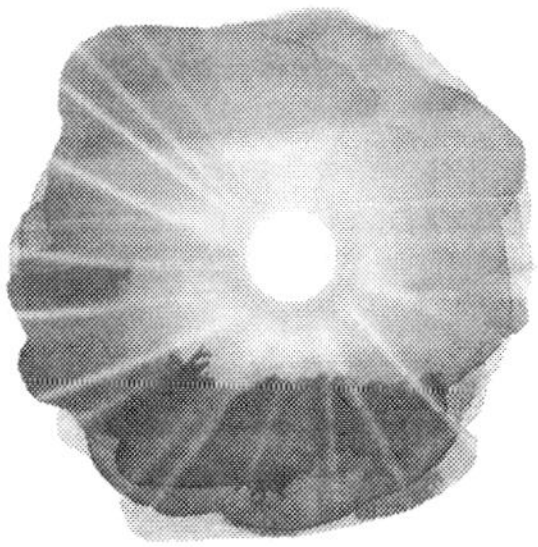

- **Step two:** *āsana* — prepare the body.

Do a short practice, emphasizing back bends and forward bends to create a *samana* effect.

- **Step three:** *prāṇāyāma* — prepare the breath.

Find a comfortable, seated position, either on the floor or in a chair. Take 12 *ujjāyī* breaths. Make the inhale and exhale the same length, to deepen the *samana* effect.

Round	Ratio in Seconds IN.HOLD.EX.HOLD	Number of Breaths
# 1	6.0.6.0	12

- **Step four:** *saṅkalpa* — state your intention.

Place your hands in *saṅkalpa mudrā* and, while looking at your chosen image, repeat your intention aloud: "I commit to completing this practice; may it show me the steps I need to take to fulfill my responsibility."

- **Step five:** *dhyāna* — meditation.

Place your hands in *cin mudrā* while continuing to gaze at your object representing the sun. Then, close your eyes and visualize the image of the sun, deepening your connection with it. Reflect until you are clear about what steps you need to take in order to fulfill your *dharma*.

- **Step six:** *samādhi* — absorption.

When you feel you have fully absorbed the clarity, sit and savor the experience. This could be several minutes or longer. Remember, this is a progressive process which will develop over time.

- **Step seven:** delinking.

When you are ready to delink from the object of meditation, take six *ujjāyī* breaths with your exhale twice as long as your inhale.

Round	Ratio in Seconds IN.HOLD.EX.HOLD	Number of Breaths
# 1	4.0.8.0	6

- **Step eight:** transition.

Maintain this focused state of mind as you perform some gentle *āsana* to reconnect with your body. Express gratitude for the clarity gained through the meditation and affirm your intention to bring it into your daily life.

Practice 4

The intention of this practice is **spirituality**, specifically, to help connect with your higher self.

- **Step one:** *dhāraṇā* — choosing an object of focus.

Choose something greater than yourself, such as a deity, nature or the universe. Place the visual representation of what you have chosen in front of you at eye level.

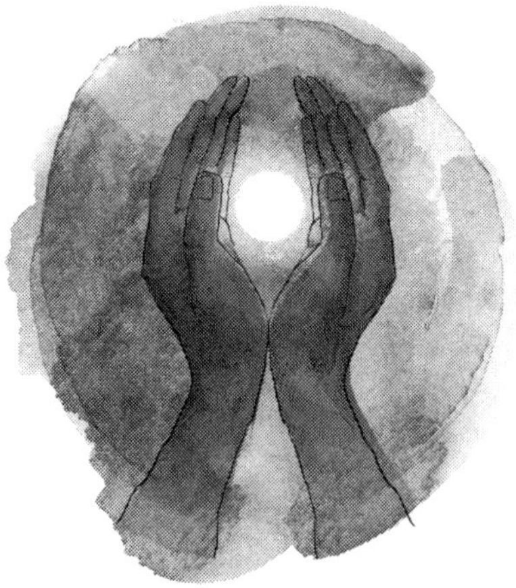

- **Step two:** *āsana* — prepare the body.

Do a short practice, emphasizing gentle forward and backbends, to help make the breath long, smooth and even, in order to produce a *samana* effect.

- **Step three:** *prāṇāyāma* — prepare the breath.

Sit either on the floor or in a chair. Do six rounds of *nāḍī śodhana* to internalize your intention.

- **Step four:** State your *saṅkalpa* — intention.

While gazing at the image, place your hands in *saṅkalpa mudrā* and repeat your intention aloud: "I commit to completing this practice; may it connect me to that which is greater than myself."

- **Step five:** *dhyāna* — meditation.

Place your hands in *dhyāna mudrā*. Gaze at the image for a while. Then, close your eyes, hold the image in your mind and feel the desired qualities of expansiveness or transcendence. Continue to deepen your connection with these qualities and observe them in yourself.

- **Step six:** *samādhi* — absorption.

When you feel you have absorbed the qualities of expansiveness or transcendence, sit and savor the experience. This can be for several minutes or longer. Remember, meditation is a profound, progressive process which will develop over time.

- **Step seven:** delinking.

When you are ready to delink from the object of meditation, take six *ujjāyī* breaths with the exhale twice as long as your inhale.

Round	Ratio in Seconds IN.HOLD.EX.HOLD	Number of Breaths
# 1	4.0.8.0	6

- **Step eight:** transition.

Maintain this focused state of mind as you perform some gentle *āsana* to reconnect with your body. Express gratitude for your meditation and the ability to bring spirituality into your daily life.

After doing any of these practices, you might feel the need for something more than *āsana* in order to transition to the next activity. If this is the case, you can try reading something inspirational, journaling, chanting or any other activity you choose.

To Sum Up:

- Three of the most common *mudrās* in meditation practice are
  1. *cin mudrā*
  2. *saṅkalpa mudrā*
  3. *dhyāna mudrā*
- The practices presented in this chapter represent four purposes for meditation:
  1. power
  2. healing
  3. *dharma*
  4. spirituality
- Meditation is a profound, progressive process. Its effects will deepen over time.
- The eight steps in a meditation practice are:
  1. *dhāraṇā* - choose an object of focus.
  2. *āsana* - prepare the body.
  3. *prāṇāyāma* - prepare the breath.
  4. *saṅkalpa* - state your intention.
  5. *dhyāna* - meditation.
  6. *samādhi* - absorption.
  7. delinking
  8. transition

CHAPTER 21

Sound and Recitation in *Yoga*

Sound is nature's universal language. The world speaks to us through the howling of the wind, the barking of a dog or our favorite piece of music. We use sound to express ourselves when conversing with a friend, singing in the shower or applauding a great performance. Hearing a song from the past often takes us to a different time and place. Whether we are soothed by the sounds of nature or overwhelmed by the cacophony of a busy city, sound has the power to affect us physically, emotionally, intellectually and spiritually.

Of all sounds, the sound of our own voice is the most influential and revealing. The quality of our voice reflects our physical health and state of mind. When we are calm, focused and healthy, our voice is clear and strong; if we are unwell or agitated, our voice gets weak, shrill or hesitant. In addition, our voice not only reflects our state of mind, it can also affect it.

In *Yoga*, we are able to affect our physical and mental energy through the use of chanting. Because chanting aloud can only be done on exhale, it promotes slower, deeper breathing. This long, smooth exhale activates the parasympathetic nervous system, leading to clearer thinking, balanced emotions and deeper relaxation.

The chants most often used in the Krishnamacharya-Desikachar lineage have their roots in Sanskrit and the *Vedic* tradition. However, sounds, syllables or words from any language or tradition can be used, providing they have positive associations for the practitioner.

Robert's story:

I had a student, an aspiring fashion designer, who was extremely timid and soft spoken. This resulted in her ideas being largely ignored by bosses and co-workers in an industry known for being fierce, outspoken and opinionated. Initially, she asked for some *Yoga* postures to increase her self-esteem. I felt that, in addition to *āsana*, chanting would also strengthen her voice and raise her confidence. At first, she was puzzled and a bit skeptical. Eventually, she agreed to add chanting to her physical practice each day before going to work. Over time, chanting dramatically strengthened her voice and boosted her self-confidence. As a result, her boss began to take her more seriously and actually listen to her ideas.

As you can see from this example, integrating sound and mental recitation with other *yogic* tools such as *āsana*, *prāṇāyāma* and meditation greatly enhances the effects of a practice.

Energetics of Sound and Recitation

The energetic effects of sound and recitation can be either *bṛṁhaṇa*, *laṅghana* or *samana*, depending on their meaning, emotional associations and vibrational quality.

Bṛṁhaṇa sounds are heating and stimulating. Chanting any word that represents heat (sun, fire, etc.) or chanting louder, faster or at a higher pitch is *bṛṁhaṇa*. Some of the many positive effects of *bṛṁhaṇa* sounds are increased vitality, mental alertness and self-confidence.

Laṅghana sounds are cooling and relaxing. Chanting any word that represents coolness (moon, water, etc.) or chanting quietly, at a lower pitch or more slowly, is *laṅghana*. Some of the effects of *laṅghana* sounds are physical relaxation, mental calmness and feelings of ease and comfort.

Samana sounds are balancing. Chanting at an even volume, medium pitch or steady tempo promotes a feeling of equilibrium. *Samana* sounds create increased physical stability, a clearer, more focused mind and greater sense of contentment.

Bīja and *Mantra*

In our tradition, *bīja* and *mantra* are the two forms of chanting most commonly used in practices to create a desired result.

Bīja (seed) are one-syllable sounds which produce a variety of effects. They are frequently the root of longer Sanskrit words, or *mantra*s, and have many meanings and associations. Energetically, sounds such as *ma*, *la* and *lum* tend to be more *laṅghana* (soothing), while *rum*, *ha* and *hum* are more *bṛṁhaṇa* (stimulating).

*Mantra*s (that which protects) are words or phrases whose meanings are often rooted in ancient teachings. Many have universal themes, such as peace, compassion or devotion, and are relevant to practitioners from any cultural or religious background. As most *mantra*s are centuries old, these powerful invocations create the desired effect through reputation as well as repetition.

These verbal formulas are often devotional in nature and are more complete thoughts than the shorter, *bīja*. According to the teachings of T. Krishnamacharya, as well as our own personal experience, *mantra*s have the potential to create a profound transformational effect at every level of our being.

Sound is a subtle, powerful tool whose application requires a great degree of individualization. Though these sounds represent universal concepts, like peace and compassion, or natural objects, like the sun and the moon, they will have different effects on each individual, depending on their own associations with them.

Traditionally chanted in Sanskrit, *mantra*s can be translated into any language appropriate to the individual. For example, "*śānti*" (peace) could be chanted "*paz*" in Spanish or "peace" in English. Once we are clear about the direction of our practice, what we want to connect with, or what we are seeking to change, we can choose to repeat the *mantra* that best suits our purpose. One example is the *mantra* "*so hum*" (I am that), which can be applied to any of the qualities we wish to embody. If we want to be more confident, for example, chanting *so hum* can represent and help cultivate our own self-confidence.

Benefits of Using Sound and Recitation in Practice

There are numerous benefits for using sound and recitation in the practice of *āsana*, *prāṇāyāma* and meditation. When applied appropriately, sound can:

- refine the breath, making it longer, smoother and more efficient.
- improve our physiological functions.
- increase our ability to focus.
- make a practice more challenging.
- boost our confidence.
- strengthen self-expression and, literally, help us find our voice.

- create a more positive emotional state.
- provide greater depth and meaning to our practice.
- keep a practice fresh, interesting and fun.

Simple Guidelines for Using Sound and Recitation in Practice

Here are some tips to help you apply sound in the most useful and effective way:

- Limit the number of different sounds in one practice.
- Use sound with *āsana* only on exhale.
- Always engage the abdomen on exhale, whether chanting aloud or silently.
- Limit the use of sound to a few postures in the practice.
- Use sound in simple standing or kneeling poses only.
- In *prāṇāyāma*, start by mentally reciting a word or simple phrase that is the length of your comfortable inhale and exhale.
- Add silent recitation on the hold after inhale and exhale, if desired.
- In meditation, begin by reciting sound aloud, then more softly, then silently.
- Transition out of meditation by reciting silently, then softly, then aloud.
- As with everything else in *Yoga*, if you aren't comfortable using sound, don't do it.

Sound and Recitation in *Āsana*

Following is a practice using simple *āsana* and the chant *so hum*. Here, we will use sound:

- in three of the seven postures
- on exhale movements
- in simple movements using your arms

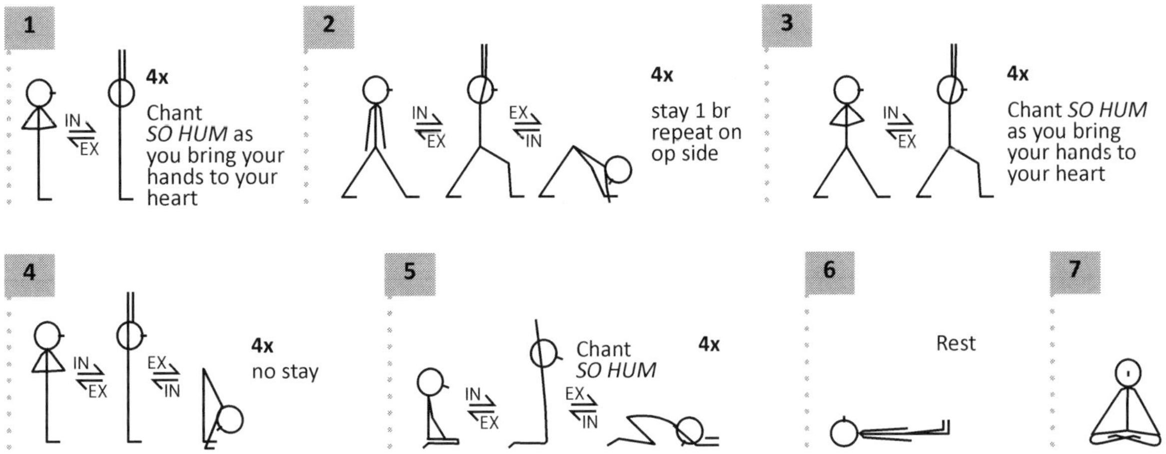

Initially, adding chant in *āsana* can create some self-consciousness with the sound of our own voice. This is a common reaction, but eventually, we become more comfortable and even come to enjoy chanting in our practice. We have found that, over time, the use of sound leads to communicating with greater self-assurance in every aspect of our lives.

Sound and Recitation in *Prāṇāyāma*

In *prāṇāyāma*, there are many ways to measure, equalize or lengthen the breath, including counting silently or using a metronome. Traditionally, because *mantras* have a fixed number of syllables, they were used as a way to measure and modify the breath.

Practice 1

The following *prāṇāyāma* practice is an example of using *mantra* to **equalize the length of the inhale and exhale** to create a *samana* effect:

1. Begin by taking several natural breaths.
2. Add *ujjāyī* to the inhale and exhale and maintain for the entire practice. Be sure to add a pause (two seconds or less) after each inhale and exhale.
3. Take four more breaths, silently reciting *so hum*, on exhale.
4. While continuing to recite *so hum* on exhale, add a silent *so hum* to your inhale and continue for four more breaths.
5. Notice how the inhale and exhale have been equalized by using the *mantra*.
6. Return to your natural breathing and observe any *samana* effects.

Practice 2

The following is an example of using *mantra* to **lengthen the exhale**, creating a *laṅghana* effect:

1. Begin by taking several natural breaths.
2. Add *ujjāyī* to the inhale and exhale and maintain for the entire practice. Remember to add a pause (two seconds or less) after each inhale and exhale.
3. Then, silently chant *so hum* on exhale and inhale. Repeat for four more breaths.
4. Continue silently chanting *so hum* on inhale. Now, to extend the exhale, add another *so hum*, chanting *so hum so hum*. Repeat for four breaths.
5. If possible, further extend the exhale by adding another *so hum*, silently chanting *so hum so hum so hum*. Repeat for four breaths.
6. Observe how changing the length of the *mantra* has extended the exhale.
7. Return to natural breathing and notice the *laṅghana* effect.

Practice 3

The next practice is an example of using *mantra* during **hold after inhale**. This will create a *bṛṁhaṇa* effect:

1. Begin by taking several natural breaths.
2. Add *ujjāyī* to both inhale and exhale and maintain for the entire practice.
3. Remember to add a pause (two seconds or less) after each inhale and exhale.
4. Add a silent *so hum* during the hold after inhale. Repeat for two breaths.
5. Add a silent *so hum so hum* during the hold after inhale. Repeat for four breaths.
6. Suspend the *mantra* from the hold after inhale and take a few *ujjāyī* breaths.
7. Return to natural breathing and notice any *bṛṁhaṇa* effects.

Sound and Recitation in Meditation

Now that you have experienced sound in *āsana* and *prāṇāyāma*, we are ready to explore *mantras* as a tool for meditation practice.

The use of sound and recitation in meditation progresses from gross to subtle and aloud to silent. Following are the guidelines for this process.

First, with eyes open, recite the sound or sounds aloud. This helps us to learn the chant, focus the mind and connect with its vibrational quality. Engage the abdomen on exhale when chanting aloud to support the sound and pace the breath.

Then, with the eyes partially closed, recite the chant softly. This will create a more inward focus and a link to what the chant represents.

Finally, recite the chant silently with the eyes fully closed. This allows us to deepen the connection to the sound itself, the feeling it creates, what it represents and all it can reveal.

Practice Using *Mantra* in Meditation:

Choosing confidence as the focus in our meditation, we will continue with *so hum*, which, in this practice represents "I am that confidence."

1. Sitting quietly with your hands in *cin mudrā*, close your eyes and visualize a person in your life whose confidence inspires you.
2. Slowly, chant *so hum* aloud five to ten times, linking to the confidence of the person you are visualizing.
3. Deepen the practice by repeating the *mantra* softly five to ten times.
4. Keeping your focus on the *mantra*, chant *so hum* silently five or more times.
5. When you feel you have absorbed the quality of confidence, sit and savor the experience. This could be for several minutes or longer.
6. When you are ready to transition, chant *so hum* **silently** 3x with eyes closed. Then chant **softly** 3x with eyes partially open. Finally, chant **aloud** 3x with eyes fully open.

A Practice Integrating *Āsana, Prāṇāyāma,* Sound and Meditation

We will now combine the elements of *āsana, prāṇāyāma,* sound and meditation in one practice, utilizing the *mantra, so hum,* with the intention of increasing confidence.

Āsana:

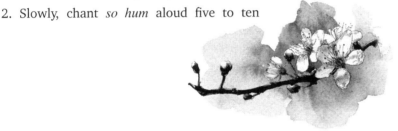

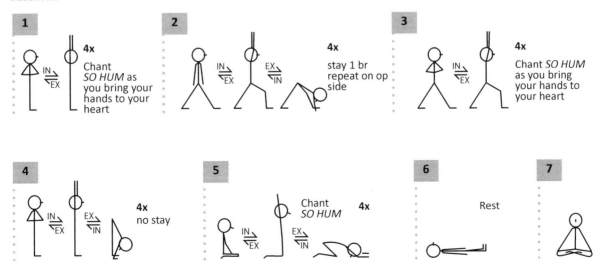

Prāṇāyāma:

8. Sitting quietly, place your hands in *cin mudra* and close your eyes. Keep them closed for the remainder of the practice.

9. Begin by taking several natural breaths.

10. Add *ujjāyī* to both the inhale and exhale. Be sure to add a pause (2 seconds or less) after each inhale and exhale. Take several breaths.

11. With all recitation done silently, chant *so hum* on inhale, taking in the feeling of confidence. Chant *so hum* on the hold after inhale, letting the quality of confidence fill your heart. Chant *so hum* on exhale, firmly established in your newfound confidence. Repeat 10 times.

12. Take a few *ujjāyī* breaths without the *mantra*.

13. Return to natural breathing and maintain your attention.

Meditation:

14. Visualize a person in your life whose confidence inspires you.

15. With the hands on your heart, chant *so hum* aloud five to ten times, linking with the confidence of the person you are visualizing.

16. Deepen the practice by repeating the *mantra* softly five to ten times, then silently for five or more times.

17. Having absorbed the qualities of confidence, sit and remain in the experience. Begin to recognize these same qualities in yourself. When you are ready, delink from the visualization. This could be several minutes or longer.

18. At the end of your meditation, inhale freely and on exhale chant *so hum* five times silently with eyes closed, then softly with eyes partly open and finally, aloud with eyes fully open.

Sit quietly and observe the effects.

19. With eyes open, do some gentle arm movements to transition. Bring this feeling of confidence into the rest of your day.

The integration of sound with *āsana*, *prāṇāyāma* and meditation helps clarify our intention, intensify the overall effect and add greater depth and meaning to any practice.

The Approach

The above practice incorporates the many tools and strategies we have discussed throughout this book. We have carefully selected and sequenced specific postures, breathing techniques and a meditation using *mantra* and *mudrā* to achieve a desired goal. This holistic approach, which integrates tools for the body, breath and mind in a single practice, is the hallmark of T. Krishnamacharya and T.K.V. Desikachar's teachings.

To Sum Up:

- Sound is nature's universal language.
- The sound of our own voice both reflects and affects our physical, psychological, emotional and spiritual states.
- Learning to use sound and recitation is a process which progresses from gross to subtle.
- Sound can have three different energetic effects: *bṛṁhaṇa*, *laṅghana* or *samana*.
- *Bīja* and *mantra* are the two forms of recitation most commonly used in practice.
- Chanting can be used to enhance the effects of *āsana*, *prāṇāyāma* and meditation.

CHAPTER 22

The Student/Teacher Relationship: The Heart of *Yoga*

On the modern *Yoga* path, we have access to a vast array of educational opportunities, including live *Yoga* *āsana* classes, websites, mobile apps and instructional books and videos. For newcomers, the journey often begins by experimenting with one or more of these options out of curiosity, for help with stress or injuries, or even recommendations from a doctor. If someone decides to try a class, they often sample several different studios, classes and instructors, looking for the right fit and experience.

After a few classes, some individuals decide *Yoga* is not for them. Others opt to go deeper, usually choosing a particular "style" or a favorite teacher. This is the first step in the process of becoming an actual student of *Yoga*, rather than just a participant. There are many benefits to group classes. These include:

- The presence of other students increases our motivation.
- A teacher leading us through a practice helps us to tune out our own thoughts.
- We enjoy the company of like-minded people.

Ultimately, however, despite their benefits, group classes can only take us so far. If we wish to apply *Yoga's* myriad of tools and strategies to our own unique, ever-changing needs, the next step is to develop a personal home practice. To insure that our practice is safe, effective and enjoyable, we need the guidance and support of an experienced teacher with whom we have a relationship. This explains why, traditionally, all adult *Yoga* students would meet privately with a teacher, from whom they would receive an individualized personal practice.

The Classic Model

There is a profound paradox at the heart of *Yoga* Philosophy. The ancient texts assure us that the answers to our most fundamental questions and solutions to our problems already exist within us. At the same time, an honest, insightful, living teacher is the most expedient and reliable way to access these inner truths.

When we are in a relationship with someone who has our best interest at heart and can mentor us, we experience increased confidence, deeper self-awareness and a greater ability to achieve our goals. A dedicated, one-on-one relationship with a teacher helps us to observe and transform our negative behaviors while supporting and deepening our strengths and virtues.

Traditionally, the student/teacher relationship had a foundation in mutual respect and an awareness of each other's roles. When a student felt they were ready, he or she would seek out a prospective teacher and express their desire to study with them. If the teacher were convinced of the student's sincerity, commitment and potential, they would consent, and the relationship would begin. The teacher, free of the student's bias and conditioning, can offer more clarity, support and an alternative perspective.

In the context of this relationship, the teacher and student would study the *Yoga Sūtras* of Patañjali, as well as a variety of other *yogic* and philosophical texts. The teacher would create a highly individualized personal practice for the student, combining all the *yogic* tools needed to improve the student's body, breath, mind and relationships.

Despite the far reaching benefits of this classical model, many modern students are unaware, hesitant or skeptical about the benefits of working privately with a teacher.

Qualities of a *Yoga* Student

- **Awareness that there is something we wish to change or achieve**. This can be anything from changing an attitude or a behavior to getting a good night's sleep or developing sharper focus.
- **Willingness to ask for help**. Though we may have been taught the importance of self-reliance, it is the ability to ask for help that ultimately leads to growth.
- **Openness to hearing a new perspective**. We must set aside the knowledge we have accumulated, as some of it may, in fact, be an impediment to change.
- **Ability to follow direction**. We must trust the teacher enough to comply with their suggestions. These might include a complete practice of *āsana, prāṇāyāma* and meditation, reading suggested texts, journaling or taking new action (*Kriya Yoga*).
- **Comfortable with a teacher and committed to practice.** It is only by practicing with enthusiasm, patience and self-reflection, that we will experience deep, positive changes. These measurable benefits will deepen our faith in both the process and the teacher over time.

Qualities of a *Yoga* Teacher

Having clarified the prerequisites for a successful student, let's examine the qualities that define an effective *Yoga* teacher. The teacher you choose should exhibit many, if not all, of the attributes described in the classical texts. According to these texts, a good teacher must be:

- **A Good Communicator.** A true teacher speaks clearly, choosing words that can be easily understood by the student. They are able to listen, empathize and hear what the student is trying to say. Then, after quietly reflecting, they give an appropriate response.
- **Mentally and emotionally stable.** A good teacher has enough self-awareness to know how to best support their students. They can empathize but they don't react, re-traumatize the student, or project their own problems or goals onto the student.
- **Honest and Ethical.** Authentic teachers live with a high level of personal integrity. They speak the truth in a way that can be heard. A great teacher is able to inspire confidence without guaranteeing success and doesn't need to boast.
- **Knowledgeable.** Good teachers are experienced in the use of many *Yogic* tools. The teacher maintains an attitude of curiosity and teachability. They are deeply interested in the true nature of things and are always willing to replace former understanding of something with a better one. An authentic teacher has an awareness of their own limitations. They know when to ask for help and when to send the student to another practitioner.

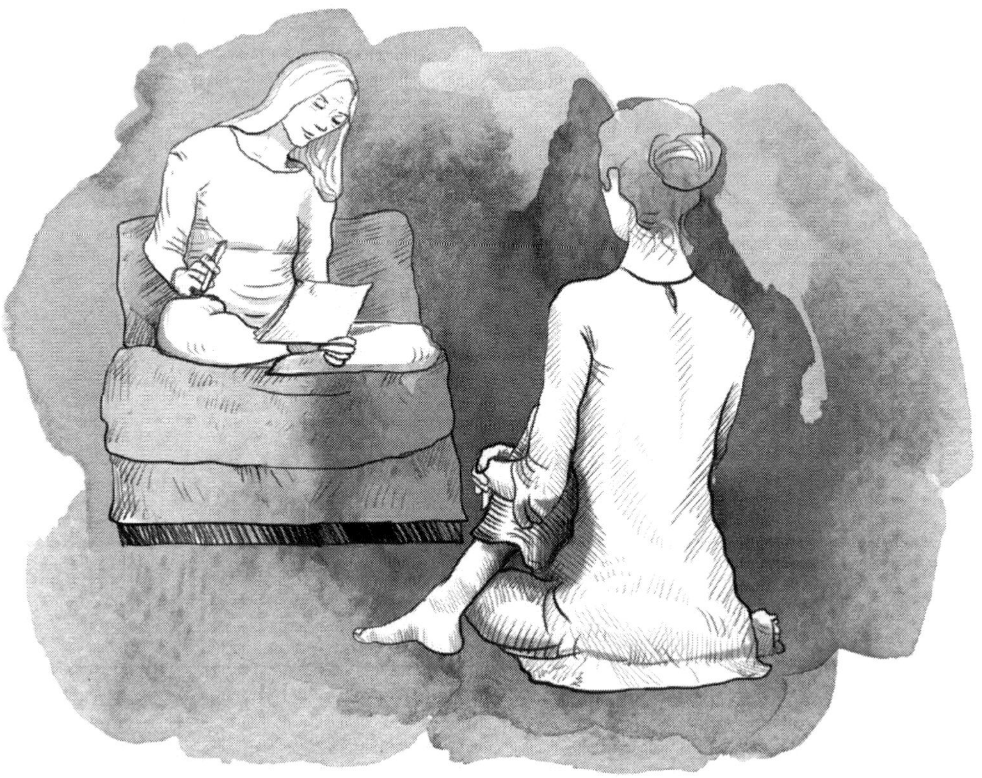

- **Faithful**. Authentic teachers possess unwavering faith in the healing system. This inspires the student and helps them to deepen their own belief in the teacher, the tools and their own ability to heal.
- **Non-Threatening.** A great teacher creates a safe learning atmosphere. They bring their positive energy and charisma to the relationship without being threatening or flirtatious.
- **Established Practitioner.** A teacher must serve as a role model. A great teacher must have a consistent, satisfying relationship with their own, ever-evolving personal practice.
- **Authoritative.** They have spent sufficient time studying and practicing with a qualified teacher who has studied with a qualified teacher.
- **Self-Disciplined.** Good teachers exercise self-control. They always maintain clear, healthy boundaries between themselves and the student. In many cases, poor boundaries are an element, if not the cause, of the student's problem(s). It is only through the teacher modeling impeccable boundaries that the student learns a new way of living with greater freedom and more control.
- **Discerning.** The true teacher is generous with their time, energy and resources but careful not to give too much, too soon. They are willing to share what they know with those who are genuinely concerned but won't waste time with those not truly interested in making changes.

Although we have just described the qualities of a true teacher, what ultimately matters is whether the teacher is right for you. If a teacher proves to be the wrong fit — even if they're highly qualified and respected — you shouldn't hesitate to continue your search for the right one.

The Gifts of Studying with a Teacher

Once you have found the right teacher, here are a few of the many benefits you can expect:

The teacher will design a personal practice based on your own individual time constraints, abilities, needs and goals. This practice will draw from the entire range of *yogic* tools including *āsana*, *prāṇāyāma*, meditation, self-study, visualization and sound.

As an educator, the teacher will add to your knowledge base as needed.

The teacher will have the ability to verify the effects and experience of your practice, continually refining or changing it to better serve your needs.

The teacher will applaud your life successes and support you through the more challenging times.

The teacher will point out your blind spots and offer additional perspectives.

This type of one-on-one instruction has been responsible for the transmission of *yogic* teachings for more than 5,000 years. Ideally, your teacher will also have a strong link with a qualified teacher. It is through this unbroken chain of relationships, rather than through simply pursuing different *yogic* styles, that *yogis* have always been identified.

Ultimately, the best teacher is someone with whom you experience an easy affinity and a natural affection, "someone around whom you breathe easier," as our teacher says. The first teacher you choose might not be the right one for you. Don't give up! If you are motivated and patient, you and your teacher will surely find each other.

To Sum Up:

- Today there are many different ways to study and gain information about *Yoga*.
- Group classes offer many benefits for beginning students.
- In the classical model, there was always a one-on-one relationship between adult students and a teacher.
- A student should be willing to choose one teacher and commit to a practice.
- A qualified teacher should be a good communicator, mentally and emotionally stable, honest and ethical, knowledgeable, faithful, non-threatening, an established practitioner, authoritative, self-disciplined and discerning.
- In a student/teacher relationship, the student can expect guidance in developing a personal practice, education, support and an alternative perspective.
- A good teacher has a strong link with their teacher and, therefore, with the entire chain of *yogic* teachings.

About the Authors

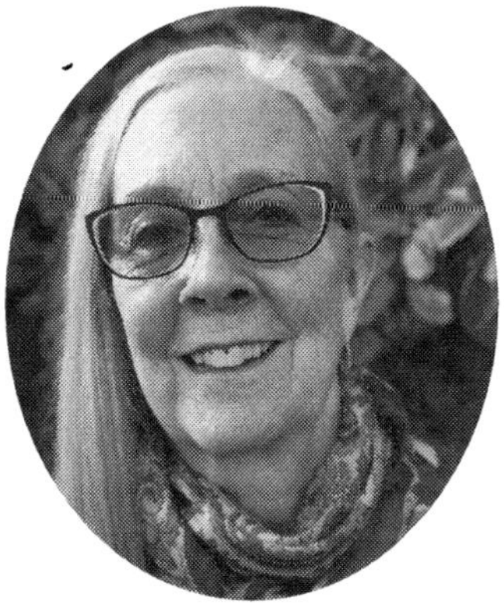

CHRISTINE DORMAIER, M.S., C-IAYT, ERYT 500 is Director of Sound*Yoga* and a Certified *Yoga* Teacher Trainer in the tradition of T. Krishnamacharya. She also holds a diploma from the American *Viniyoga* Institute as a *Yoga* therapist. Chris teaches ongoing *Yoga Sūtra* study and therapeutic group *Yoga* classes. As a *Yoga* therapist she applies *Yoga* principles in developing practices that support and meet the needs of individuals who strive for better health and a happier, more balanced lifestyle. She produced Strong Bones *Yoga*, an instructional video for building bone density and the prevention of osteoporosis. Chris continues her studies with Sonia Nelson in Santa Fe, New Mexico.

Chris can be contacted at info@soundyoga.com

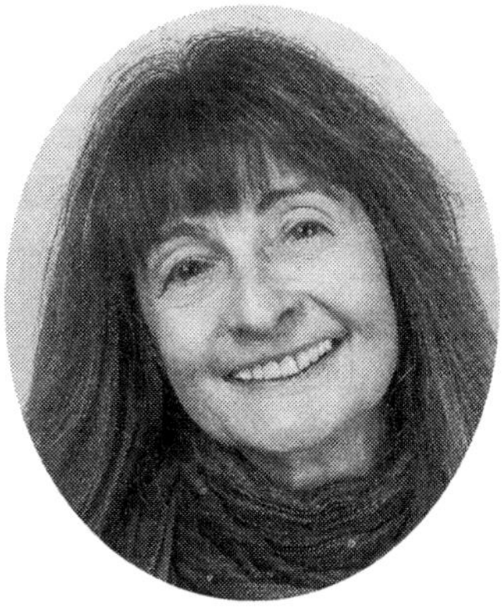

FRAN UBERTINI, ERYT 500, C-IAYT, is director of *Yoga* for Well-Being™, a Certified *Yoga* Teacher Trainer in the tradition of T. Krishnamacharya and a graduate of the American *Viniyoga* Institute as a *Yoga* Therapist. After exploring various *Yoga* traditions, she discovered T.K.V. Desikachar's classic The Heart of *Yoga*, which launched her dedicated *Yoga* studies. She has been teaching *Yoga*, training teachers and working as a *Yoga* therapist for over 20 years in this tradition.

Fran works nationally, training teachers and mentoring them in their continuing education. As a *Yoga* therapist she works with clients to help them create and maintain health and well-being in their lives. She continues her studies and long-term relationship with Sonia Nelson in Santa Fe, New Mexico.

Fran can be contacted at franubertini@yahoo.com

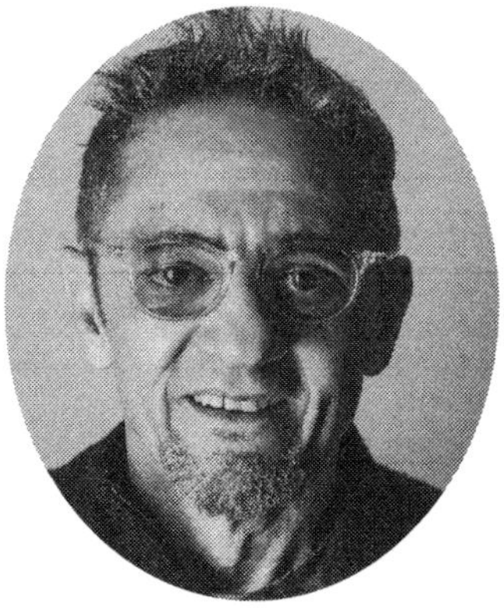

ROBERT BIRNBERG has been a student of *Yoga* for over 40 years. He has studied with T.K.V. Desikachar, his family and various senior teachers for over 25 years. Robert interned at the T. Krishnamacharya *Yoga* Mandiram (KYM), an institution regarded internationally for *Yoga* education and therapy. He is a Certified *Yoga* Teacher Trainer in the tradition of T. Krishnamacharya. Robert teaches private, therapeutic *Yoga*, presents ongoing *Yoga Sutras* study groups, and trains teachers in the U.S. and abroad. He is on the faculty of Loyola Marymount's *Yoga* Therapy Program and is a certified Positive Psychology Coach.

He specializes in relationship coaching and the treatment of addiction. He lectures internationally and has been published in *Yoga* periodicals.

Robert can be contacted at longexhale@mac.com

Sanskrit Pronunciation Guide

GUTTURAL
(pronounced from the throat)

vowels	a	as in cut
	ā	as in father
plain	k	as in kid
	g	as in get
aspirate	kh	as in sinkhole
	gh	as in leghorn
	h	as in hear
nasal	ṅ	as in oncology

PALATAL
(pronounced from the palate)

vowels	i	as in bit
	ī	as in bead
plain	c	as in churn
	j	as in justice
aspirate	ch	as in coachhorse
	jh	as in hedgehog
semivowel	y	as in yes
sibilant	ś	as in shirt

RETROFLEX
(pronounced with the tip of your tongue curled up)

vowels	ṛ	as in sabre
	ṝ	as in grin
plain	ṭ	as in dart
	ḍ	as in order
aspirate	ṭh	as in carthorse
	ḍh	as in fordham
nasal	ṇ	as in send
semivowel	r	as in run
sibilant	ṣ	as in bush

DENTAL
(pronounced with the tip of the tongue against the upper teeth)

vowels	ḷ	as in label
plain	t	as in think
	d	as in day
aspirate	th	as in withheld
	dh	as in buddha
nasal	n	as in spoon
semivowel	l	as in loose
sibilant	s	as in sand

LABIAL
(pronounced with the lips)

vowels	u	as in pull
	ū	as in cool
plain	p	as in pole
	b	as in big
aspirate	ph	as in uphill
	bh	as in abhor
nasal	m	as in moon

GUTTERAL AND PALATAL

vowels	e	as in they
	ai	as in aisle

GUTTERAL AND LABIAL

vowels	o	as in so
	au	as in wow

DENTAL AND LABIAL

semivowel	v	as in vice

NASAL

ṁ (ṃ) or ṅ makes the preceding vowel nasal

ASPIRATE

ḥ makes the preceding vowel aspirate

Glossary of Sanskrit Terms

A

abhiniveśa: any fear that prevents us from living a rich, full life, ultimately the fear of dying; one of the five *kleśas*

adhomukha svanāsana: downward-facing dog pose

Ādhyātmika Krama: one of five methodologies of *Yoga* practices offered by T. Krishnamacharya, a deeply contemplative practice that emphasize meditation, prayer and ritual to achieve inner peace and self-realization

agni: digestive fire

ahiṁsā: espect for life and kindness for all living things; root principle of the five *yamas*

Amarakośa: an eighth century thesaurus of Sanskrit terms

ānandamaya: In the *Pañca Maya* Model: our capacity for joy

annamaya: In the *Pañca Maya* Model: our anatomy or physical structure

anuloma ujjāyī: a breathing technique using *ujjāyī* on the inhale and the alternate nostril on the exhale

apānāsana: lower abdomen pose

apāna vāyu: lifeforce responsible for downward movement in the body

aparigraha: not grasping; the fifth *yama*

ardha: half

ardha śalabhāsana: half-locust pose

ardha utkaṭāsana: half-chair pose

ardha uttānāsana: half-forward bend pose

āsana: the physical postures; the third of the eight limbs

asmitā: ego, confused self-image; one of the five *kleśas*

Aṣṭāṅga Yoga: Patañjali's eight limbs. A holistic model that offers guidelines for balanced living in the areas of relationships, lifestyle, body, breath, senses and the mind.

asteya: being honest in our actions; the third *yama*

atharva: one of the four books of the *Vedas*

avidyā: misperceiving reality; the root *kleśa*

Āyurveda: science of life, a system of traditional Indian medicine

B

baddhakoṇāsana: bound-angle pose

bekāsana: frog pose

Bhagavad Gītā: Song of the Beloved; a sacred text of Hinduism and a primary reference for *Yoga*

bhāvana: the process of visualization used to clarify values and help us move toward our goals.

bhujaṅgāsana: cobra pose

bīja: seed

brahmacarya: practicing moderation, control and not allowing distractions to get in the way of achieving our highest goal; the fourth *yama*

brahmāsana: supreme god pose

bṛṁhaṇa: to increase, expand, heat and energize

C

cakravākāsana: ruddy goose pose, a slight back arch

chale vāte, chalaṁ cittaṁ: "As the breath goes, so the mind goes" from the *Haṭha Yoga Pradīpikā*

caturānga daṇḍāsana: four-limb stick pose

cin mudrā: a hand gesture in which the index finger and thumb touch to form a circle

Cikitsā Krama: one of five kinds of *Yoga* methodologies offered by T. Krishnamacharya, a *Yoga* therapy that can be implemented at any stage of life

D

daṇḍāsana: seated stick pose

Darśanas: ways of looking at life; a collection of six philosophical systems *(Nyāya, Vaiśeṣika, Sāṃkhya, Mīmāṃsā, Vedānta* and *Yoga)* that offer six distinct paths to the common goal of identifying and reducing suffering

deśa: place or location (climate, altitude and general ambience); one of Patañjali's three components of practice

dhāraṇā: choosing an object, the first step in the process of meditation; the sixth of the eight limbs

dharma: one's roles and responsibilities in life

dhanurāsana: bow pose

dhyāna: meditation or continuous focused attention; one of five definitions of *Yoga* offered by T. Krishnamacharya and the seventh of the eight limbs

dīrgha: long; one of Patañjali's two qualities of breath

duḥkha: suffering, discomfort

dveṣa: unreasonable aversion to that which once caused us discomfort or reminds of us of something that did; one of the five *kleśas*

dvipādapīṭham: bridge pose

G

Gheraṇḍa Saṁhitā: a classical *Yoga* text

guṇas: degrees or rates of change; the three energetic qualities of all matter (*prakṛti*)

H

Haṭha Yoga: physical aspect of *Yoga* practice, classically defined as, merging the two energies, *iḍā* and *piṅgala*, heating and cooling to the center of the spine.'

Haṭha Yoga Pradīpikā: a classical *Yoga* text

I

icchā: wish, degree of commitment, intensity of desire

iḍā: left channel; one of the *nāḍīs*

īśvarapraṇidhāna: an attitude that results in the ability to focus on the quality of our actions rather than on the outcome; the third component of *Kriyā Yoga;* the fifth *niyama*

J

jānuśīrṣāsana: head to knee pose

jānuśīrṣāsana pārśva bheda: head to knee pose with lateral variation

jaṭhara parivṛtti (ekapāda): one-legged twist

jaṭhara parivṛtti (parivṛtti): two-legged twist

jaṭhara parivṛtti (pārśva): twist with lateral variation

K

kaivalya: lasting freedom, one of the goals of *Yoga*

kāla: time (time of day, length of practice); one of Patañjali's three components of practice

kleśas: the five inherent tendencies in the mind that are the source of all suffering,

Kramas: the five methodologies developed and taught by Krishnamacharya, based on the *Vedic* stage-of-life model, as well as on his extensive knowledge of *Āyurveda* and the *Yoga Sūtras*

Kriyā Yoga: *Yoga* of Action, *Tapas*, *Svādhyāya* and *Īśvarapraṇidhāna*

L

laṅghana: to reduce, relax and cool

M

Mahābhārata: an epic Indian story which includes the *Bhagavad Gītā*

mahāmudrā: great seal pose

mala: the accumulated waste of poor diet; undigested experiences

manomaya: In the *Pañca Maya* Model: our cognitive mind

mantra: word or phrase; that which protects

ardha matsyendrāsana: seated twist named after the sage, Matsyendra

maya: something that permeates

Mīmāṃsā: one of the *Darśanas*

mṛgi mudrā: a closed hand gesture with pinkie, ring finger and thumb extended

mudrās: hand gestures with a symbolic meaning that direct the energy of the body and activities of the mind in a particular direction

N

nāḍī śodhana: a breathing technique using alternate nostril breathing on both inhale and exhale

nāḍīs: subtle energy channels that run throughout the human body

nāvāsana: boat pose

nava śarīra saṁskāra: new body patterns

niyamas: lifestyle attitudes and behavioral guidelines which help to cultivate discipline and overcome our innate resistance to change; the second of the eight limbs

Nyāya: one of the *Darśanas*

P

padmāsana: full lotus pose

pañca: five

pañca maya: *Yoga*'s subtle anatomy describing five inter-connected aspects or dimensions of the individual

parivṛtti: to revolve or twist; twisting classification of *āsana*

pārśva: side or lateral; side stretching classification of *āsana*

pārśva uttānāsana: one-sided forward bend

paścimatāna: stretching the west; forward bend classification of *āsana*

paścimatānāsana: seated forward bend

piñca-mayūrāsana: feathered peacock pose

piṅgala: right channel; one of the *nāḍīs*

pradhānāṅga: the part of a practice where we arrive at the goal

prakṛti: 1. the material world, whose form is constantly changing. 2. the ideal form of the posture

prāṇa: life force or vital energy

Prāṇa/Agni/Mala: the holistic, energetic model upon which *āsana* and *prāṇāyāma* are based

prāṇamaya: In the *Pañca Maya* Model: our physiological functions

prāṇa vāyu: lifeforce responsible for all that we take in

prāṇāyāma: control and regulation of the breath; the fourth of the eight limbs

prasārita pāda uttānāsana: wide feet forward bend

pratikriyāsana: counterposes

pratyāhāra: the proper use of the senses as an instrument of our consciousness, rather than a distracting force; the fifth of the eight limbs

puruṣa: spirit; the formless, unchanging, individual consciousness at the core of our being; one of the two components of *Sāṃkhya*

pūrvāṅga: the first part of a practice, preparation

for the goal posture

***pūrvātāna**:* stretching the east: backbend classification of *āsana*

***pūrvātānāsana**:* backbending pose

R

***rāga**:* excessive craving for something which once brought us pleasure but no longer does so; one of the five *kleśas*

***rajas**:* intense and dynamic quality of change; the first *guṇa*

***rajas*ic**: expressing the qualities of rajas

***Rakṣaṇa Krama**:* one of five methodologies offered by T. Krishnamacharya in which practices are designed to protect the physical body, maintain health and prevent disease

***Rg**:* the first of four books of the *Vedas*

***ṛṣi**:* wise man

S

***śakti**:* energy

***śalabhāsana**:* locust pose

***Sāma**:* the second of four books of the *Vedas*

***samādhi**:* complete absorption in the object of meditation; the eighth of the eight limbs

samana: to equalize, balance

***samāna vāyu**:* lifeforce responsible for digestion

***samasthiti**:* equal or balanced; classification of *āsana* in which the spine is extended

***saṁgati**:* to link two objects together; one of five definitions of *Yoga* offered by T. Krishnamacharya

***Sāṃkhya**:* the philosophical system of evolution on which *Yoga* is based; one of the *Darśanas*

***saṁtoṣa**:* contentment; the second *niyama*

saṅkalpa: intention

***sannāha**:* the preparation taken before beginning a journey toward a goal; one of five definitions of *Yoga* offered by T. Krishnamacharya

***sarvaṅgāsana**:* shoulderstand

***sattva**:* change that is harmonious, balanced and sustainable; the third *guṇa*

***sattvic**:* expressing the qualities of *sattva*

***satya**:* telling the truth or being honest in our communication; the second *yama*

***śauca**:* cleanliness, purity, proper physical hygiene; the first *niyama*

***śavāsana**:* corpse pose

***śānti**:* peace

***siddhāsana**:* accomplished seated pose

***Śikṣaṇa**:* the perfection of the form

***Śikṣaṇa Krama**:* one of five methodologies of *Yoga* practice offered by T. Krishnamacharya, with emphasis on mastery of the classical postures

***śīrṣāsana**:* headstand

***śītalī**:* controlling the breath by curling the tongue like a straw and inhaling through it

***śītkārī**:* inhaling with the tip of the tongue pressed against the back of the teeth

***Śiva Sūtras**:* a classical *Yoga* text

***śraddhā**:* faith and conviction

***Sṛṣṭi Krama**:* one of the five methodologies of *Yoga* practice offered by T. Krishnamacharya, with the emphasis on developing strength, flexibility, confidence and discipline

***sthira**:* a firm body, steady breath and focused, alert mind

***sukha**:* a comfortable body, smooth breathing and a mind at ease

***sukhāsana**:* easy, seated pose

***sūkṣma**:* subtle, smooth; one of the defining qualities of *prāṇāyāma*

***supta baddhakoṇāsana**:* lying bound angle pose

suṣumṇā: the main, central channel of the *nāḍīs*

sūtra: is a form of writing characterized by short phrases or aphorisms with a depth of meaning

svādhyāya: self-study, self-reflection; the second component of *Kriyā Yoga;* the fourth *niyama*

T

taḍākamudrā: interlocking hands posture

tāḍāsana: mountain pose

tamas: heaviness, dullness and resistance to change; the second *guṇa*

tamasic: expressing the qualities of *tamas*

tapas: new, often challenging, behaviors aimed at refinement; the first component of *Kriyā Yoga*; the third *niyama*

U

udāna vāyu: lifeforce responsible for all upward movement in the body

ujjāyī: breathing technique in which we breathe through the nostrils with a slight constriction in the back of the throat

upaviṣṭakoṇāsana: seated wide-legged pose

ūrdhva dhanurāsana: upward bow pose

ūrdhva prasāritapādāsana: upward extended-leg pose

Upaniṣads: to sit near; a vedic text offering a broad range of theoretical teachings and practical tools for living

upāya: the ability to do something tomorrow that was formerly not possible; one of five definitions of *Yoga* offered by T. Krishnamacharya

ūrdhva mukha śvāsāsana: upward-facing dog pose

uṣṭrāsana: camel pose

utkaṭāsana: chair pose

uttaraṅga: the final part of a practice where we create a smooth transition to the next activity

utthita pārśvakoṇāsana: standing side-angle pose

utthita trikoṇāsana parivṛtti: standing triangle twisting pose

utthita trikoṇāsana (Pārśva): standing triangle pose

uttānāsana: standing forward bend

V

Vaiśeṣika: one of the six *Darśanas*

vajrāsana: kneeling diamond pose

vayah: age, stage of life

vāyu: wind, air, breath

vyāna vāyu: life-force responsible for circulation in the body

Vedas: knowledge or wisdom; India's ancient teachings "received" by great sages in their meditations.

Vedānta: one of the six *Darśanas*

Vijñānamaya: In the *Pañca Maya* Model: our individual personality, character and values

vikṛti: the actual form of a posture an individual is capable of achieving on any given day

viloma ujjāyī: a breathing technique using *ujjāyī* breathing on the exhale and the alternate nostril on the inhale

vinyāsas: a series of *Yoga* poses strung together

vinyāsa krama: small logical steps toward a chosen aim

viparīta: active reversal; classification of inverted postures

viparītakaraṇī: half shoulder stand

vīrabhadrāsana: warrior pose

viśeṣa: special or unusual; a category of postures that includes arm and leg balances

vṛtti: activities

vṛkṣāsana: tree pose

Y

Yajur: the third of the four books of the *Vedas*

yamas: relationship guidelines; the first of the eight limbs

Yoga: to join two or more things together or to

link; one of the six Darśanas, wisdom teachings for enhancing personal growth and transformation

Yoga Makaranda*:* a classical *Yoga* text

Yoga Sūtras*:* Patañjali's classic *Yoga* text

Yoga Yājñavalkya*:* a classical *Yoga* text

yogi*:* one who practices *Yoga*

yogic*:* referring or pertaining to *Yoga*

yukti*:* the skillful use of appropriate tools or strategies to achieve a desired result; one of five definitions of *Yoga* offered by T. Krishnamacharya

Index

87927537R00086

Made in the USA
Middletown, DE
06 September 2018